Self-Disciplined Dieter

How to Lose Weight
and Become Healthy
Despite Cravings
and Weak Willpower

By Martin Meadows

Download another Book for Free

I want to thank you for buying my book and offer you another book (just as valuable as this book), *Grit: How to Keep Going When You Want to Give Up*, completely free.

Visit the link below to receive it:

http://www.profoundselfimprovement.com/selfdisciplineddieter

In *Grit*, I'll share with you exactly how to stick to your goals according to peak performers and science.

In addition to getting *Grit*, you'll also have an opportunity to get my new books for free, enter giveaways, and receive other valuable emails from me.

Again, here's the link to sign up:

http://www.profoundselfimprovement.com/selfdisciplineddieter

Table of Contents

Prologue

You would like to lose weight despite the temptations, cravings, discouragement, and other common emotions and challenges associated with dieting. Either you've tried before and failed, or it's your first time and you have heard from your friends and family how hard it is to stay self-disciplined.

Maybe you could simply use a boost of self-discipline to stick to your diet for a while longer to shed off those final pounds.

Self-discipline and its cousin willpower have a strong influence on whether you succeed or fail with your diet.

This book will provide answers and advice to help you succeed when dieting – despite all of the obstacles that are so hard to overcome, and make the pursuit of losing weight a demanding challenge.

We will cover the 5 most important realizations for dieters that will help you start your diet on the right note. We'll dig into the topic of cravings and how to deal with them in a smart way. We'll also cover some scientifically-based ways to improve satiety to make dieting less challenging.

You'll learn how to part ways with unhealthy food forever (or just stop eating it regularly, as the goal is not to turn you into a person eating salads exclusively without any occasional indulgences), deal with the most common excuses and rationalizations of dieters (which are in fact problems with self-discipline) and finally, help you design a more self-disciplined life in a more holistic way.

As an author of personal development books – including books about self-discipline and persistence, I'm familiar with the vicious cycle of self-change. Few things make people more discouraged than trying over and over and getting no results.

With this book, I hope to help you break this cycle and finally achieve the change you so desperately want in your life. Things can get better, and I'm here to give you a helping hand.

Disclaimer: as in all my books, yet again I emphasize an important point – I'm not a doctor or a psychologist by training and am not qualified in any way to make life decisions for you. You should consult a trained individual about every piece of advice you want to use; especially when making decisions regarding your health.

Note: I came up with the idea for this book while writing a subchapter about this topic in my previous book, *Daily Self-Discipline*. Some paragraphs from my old work were adapted and expanded upon for this book.

Chapter 1: 5 Important Realizations to Boost Your Self-Discipline on a Diet

As much knowledge as there is about dieting, few people are aware of some key characteristics that can either make or break your resolve. Understanding some of the most important peculiarities about dieting and their effect on your self-discipline can be of tremendous help.

In this chapter, we'll cover some of these surprising facts as well as the proper attitude you need to succeed. Without this basic, fundamental knowledge, you'll struggle much more than you need to.

Dieting Takes a Lot of Time – Set the Right Expectations

Well, duh, right? Not really. Most people underestimate how long it takes to lose excess weight, and it's one of the most common reasons they fail.

A rule of thumb says you need an energy deficit of 3500 kcal to lose a pound of fat[i]. To establish a weekly deficit of 3500 kcal, you need to have a daily deficit of 500 calories.

According to the national survey data mentioned in the 2010 Dietary Guidelines for Americans, the average reported calorie intake among women and men older than age 19 years are estimated to be 1,785 and 2,640 calories per day[ii].

However, a 2003 study on the differences between estimated caloric requirements and self-reported caloric intake among women shows that subjects underreported their caloric intake by about 25%[iii].

In other words, the cited 1,785 and 2,640 calories are actually closer to 2,230 calories for females and 3,300 calories for males. Given that the U.S. Department of Agriculture reports a sedentary female aged 18+ requires 1,600 to 2,000 calories and a male aged 18+ requires 2,000 to 2,400 calories[iv] a day, there's an average daily surplus of 230 to 630 calories for females and 900 to 1,300 calories for men.

To find out your individual needs, you can calculate your Basal Metabolic Rate (BMR) by using the Harris Benedict Equation formula to determine your total daily energy expenditure (calories you need to maintain your current weight). Then you can subtract a specific amount of calories from your daily diet, say, 500 calories, to achieve a deficit of 3500 calories a week. Google "BMR calculator" or "Harris Benedict Equation" to find useful tools to help you calculate your own total daily energy expenditure.

Be aware of the fact that calorie intake is higher for overweight and obese individuals. The average person who wants to go on a diet might have a daily surplus of 1,000 calories for women and over 1,500 calories for men. Now add the 500 calories a day deficit for the diet, and you're cutting 2,000 calories off your daily intake, day in, day out, just to lose a pound of fat a week.

Consequently, you can't revert years of unhealthy eating habits within days or weeks. People who don't realize this fact are most likely to give up. It's tempting to give up after three months when you realize there are still several months left – if not more than a year – to achieve your ideal weight.

If, however, you set the right expectations in the beginning, you'll greatly reduce the temptation to give up. You'll be prepared, and that will boost your self-discipline while reducing the discouragement.

If we focus on sustainable weight loss long term, losing a pound of fat a week is a safe number. This means about 4 pounds a month and 48 pounds a year. Calculate how much weight you want to lose and how long it will take you according to these numbers, not to the unrealistic claims in articles about miracle diets.

With this knowledge, you can avoid the false hope syndrome (setting unrealistic expectations and failing only to begin yet again with another set of unrealistic expectations) that leads to frequent, unsuccessful and frustrating attempts to change[v]. You can start your diet on the right note, with the right expectations. If you're prepared from the beginning that it will take you several months or over a year to achieve your goal, you'll need much less willpower to stick to your diet.

It's Not About Only Self-Discipline and Willpower

Self-discipline is one of several pieces of the puzzle for success when dieting. Self-discipline – continuously choosing deferred gratification over an instant reward – is the first tool to stick to a diet. I cover a lot of the details regarding building powerful self-discipline in my books *How to Build Self-Discipline* and *Daily Self-Discipline*.

Willpower is a similar concept. While most people use willpower and self-discipline interchangeably, I like to describe self-discipline as something that applies to the general long-term attitude (e.g. your daily routines), while willpower is your self-control ability you use in specific situations (e.g. resisting a piece of a cake).

However, you can't expect to succeed with only sheer willpower or self-discipline. In some cases, you'll lack both of these tools, and if you don't have the other three –the right motivation, positive mindset, and established habits – you'll fail.

For instance, your willpower can fail when you eat too much and feel guilty. You become prone to the "screw it, I messed up" thoughts that will lead to further cheating. Entering a vicious cycle is almost a guarantee until you use the other tools.

A positive mindset is the first of these tools. If you think from the beginning that you'll fail, then no amount of self-discipline will help you escape this self-fulfilling prophecy. Moreover, thinking that slip ups are fine as long as you keep going can help you deal with setbacks in a sensible way.

Having the right motivation – the second of these tools – can aid as well. A twenty-something male trying to lose weight to attract women will have a weaker resolve than a fifty-something female that has to lose weight or have a guaranteed heart attack.

Last but not least, you need established habits. If you do a particular activity automatically (say, drink a cup of coffee in the morning), you don't need any amount of willpower to keep repeating this behavior on a daily basis.

If you develop a habit of eating healthy on a daily basis, then, you'll still return to your default behavior even when you face obstacles. That's why developing proper habits is another key to achieve success – even if you lose willpower for a short period of time, your habits will be there to support you.

Studies have shown it takes anywhere from 18 days to 254 days to form a new habit[vi]. On average, it takes 66 days to make a new behavior automatic.

Each day you repeat the habit you intend to make a part of your daily schedule, you need less discipline to make it stick. We'll cover how to stick to your habit long enough to make it an ingrained habit in detail later.

Your Diet Matters Little (and Sometimes a Lot)

Dr. David Katz and Stephanie Meller at Yale University's Prevention Research Center compared various popular diets such as a low carb diet, low fat diet, low glycemic diet, Mediterranean diet, mixed/balanced (DASH) diet, Paleolithic diet, vegan diet, and elements of other common weight loss diets[vii].

The conclusion of their research is that every diet is associated with health promotion and disease prevention as long as it's "of minimally processed foods close to nature, predominantly plants."

In other words, as long as you choose a diet that focuses in one way or another on eating unprocessed foods and avoiding highly-processed ones, you'll be fine. Whether you'll choose a low carb diet, a Paleo diet, DASH diet, or any other popular diet, you can expect similar results as long as you stick to it.

The only thing that makes a difference when picking a diet is its impact on your self-discipline. While all of the mentioned diets can work, it doesn't mean all will work well for you.

For some people, a low carb diet is a nightmare because they feel too restricted if they can't eat any of their favorite high-carb foods. For other people, a Paleo diet and the exclusion of all kinds of grains is too challenging. Before committing to a diet, ask yourself which one sounds too restrictive to you and which one sounds bearable or even easy.

I used the slow-carb diet[viii] for my own weight loss because I liked its simplicity and the ability to enjoy my favorite foods on a weekly basis.

Later on, I made some changes to it and then abandoned it once I reached my target weight and wanted to transition to something more sustainable with fewer restrictions. However, it did its job during the weight loss period without challenging my willpower too much.

It was the right fit for me. A vegan diet, for example, wouldn't have been because I would find it too difficult to stop eating eggs and dairy.

Pick your diet carefully, but don't think about it too much in terms of effectiveness. Instead, focus on how easy or difficult it sounds to maintain for the next few months (or any other period to reach your target weight you've calculated with the 3500 calories per pound of fat rule).

Permanent Change Is Not about Dieting

Far too many people believe that everything will be fine and dandy if they only go on a three-month diet, lose a few pounds, and then go back to their old eating habits. I'm sorry to say, but that's not how it works.

If you want permanent changes, you have to change your life permanently. A diet (including more restrictive ones) can help you reach your target weight, but it's only the first step toward optimal health.

Once you finish your weight loss diet, it will be time to make other permanent changes to your eating habits. The first few months of your diet, when you're on a calorie deficit, will be different than the diet you'll follow once you lose excess weight and want to go back to the maintenance level of calories. If you think of your diet in terms of "well, I'll just stick to it for a few months, lose what pounds I have to lose and then go back to eating pizza for breakfast," you'll only be disappointed because you'll quickly regain your weight (and then some).

We'll discuss proper habits and building your new lifestyle in Chapter 5 and 6. For now, just remember that if you're not committed to making permanent changes in your life (and yes, that includes either lessening or no longer eating certain foods), you might as well close this book now and forget about dieting because it won't change anything in the grand scheme of things.

Extreme Diets Can Be More Effective (And Boost Your Willpower)

Contrary to popular belief, as long as you're overweight or obese, rapid weight loss can be more effective than slow weight loss (it's not beneficial for the elderly[ix] or lean people[x], though).

A 2000 review conducted by Danish researchers showed that "greater initial weight loss induced without changes in lifestyle (e.g. liquid formula diets or anorectic drugs) improves long-term weight maintenance, providing it is followed by a 1–2 years integrated weight maintenance programme"[xi].

A 2001 review by a Dutch scientist has shown that "there is evidence that a greater initial weight loss using VLCDs (very-low-calorie diets) with an active follow-up weight-maintenance program, including behavior therapy, nutritional education and exercise, improves weight maintenance"[xii].

Researchers conducting a 2010 study on 262 middle-aged obese women also found that there are "both short- and long-term advantages to fast initial weight loss. Fast weight losers obtained greater weight reduction and long-term maintenance, and were not more susceptible to weight regain than gradual weight losers"[xiii].

Finally, a 2014 Australian study on the rate of weight loss affecting long-term weight management has shown that "the rate of weight loss does not affect the proportion of weight regained within 144 weeks"[xiv]. In other words, there was no difference between the gradual weight loss and the rapid weight loss group in terms of who has regained it.

As the scientists concluded, "These findings are not consistent with present dietary guidelines which recommend gradual over rapid weight loss, based on the belief that rapid weight loss is more quickly regained."

If you want to start your diet with a boost of motivation and increase your willpower for the future, consider a rapid weight loss diet that will help you shed off a few pounds in the first few weeks.

Just remember that the goal is to rapidly lose fat, not muscle or water weight through dehydrating yourself – for this reason, make sure you have enough protein and water in your diet. Once the diet becomes too difficult to maintain, make it less drastic (increase your daily calorie consumption and/or include certain food groups that were banned before but are healthy).

If you're an impatient person, when you see such quick results, you'll be more determined to keep going than if you were to start slowly. If you're fine with a more unhurried progress, a slow and steady approach will work, too.

5 IMPORTANT REALIZATIONS TO BOOST YOUR SELF-DISCIPLINE ON A DIET: QUICK RECAP

1. Dieting takes a lot of time. If you don't set the right expectations, you're bound to fail. Calculate how much weight you can lose with the rule of a deficit of 3500 calories a week to burn a pound of fat. Accept that slow loss is the most likely outcome – and not the results suggested by the creators of miracle diets. Use a BMR calculator and the Harris Benedict Equation to find out your individual daily energy expenditure and then calculate your weekly deficit.

2. When dieting, you can't rely on your willpower alone. If you don't have the right motivation and a positive attitude, it will be hard to keep pushing when everything goes wrong. Develop positive habits to support your willpower. You'll repeat them automatically even if your willpower fails.

3. As long as your diet focuses on whole foods, it doesn't matter whether you follow a paleo diet, a low-

carb diet, or a low-glycemic diet. All of these diets can lead to success. What matters is the diet/dieter fit. If a diet you want to follow is overly restrictive for your personal situation (say, it forbids eating fruits and you love eating them), it will likely lead to a failure. Choose a diet that fits your eating habits the most and that you can maintain for the long term.

4. Permanent change is not about dieting. If you approach dieting as a short-term fix (and then you want to go back to your old unhealthy eating habits), you'll never make lasting changes in your life. It's only when you combine dieting with developing proper, permanent eating habits you can achieve lifelong success.

5. Rapid weight loss diets can be more successful than regular diets if you're overweight or obese. If you're impatient and likely to give up if you don't see quick results, consider following a more extreme diet for a few weeks. Once you see quick, noticeable results, you'll get motivated to keep going (even when you eventually switch to a safer, slower diet).

Chapter 2: How to Deal with Cravings

No matter if you have a strong resolve or not, you'll experience cravings at some point during your diet.

Overpowering cravings can lead to unscheduled, uncontrollable gorging on unhealthy foods that frequently leads to guilt and the abrupt end of the diet.

How can you improve your self-control and handle cravings with more ease? Is it even possible at all? In this chapter we'll explore the answers to these questions.

The Essence of a Craving

Cravings are usually triggered by a certain cue and followed by a specific action (your habit).

If you crave chocolate, it can be because you saw someone eating a chocolate bar. The habit that follows is buying chocolate for yourself.

If you can't help but think about eating pizza after driving past a pizzeria, then that's your cue. The habit is go stop by and order pizza.

If you think about ice cream after eating dinner, then maybe your cue is that you're used to eating a dessert and your body is trained to expect it at a specific hour.

A signal (cue) leads to a temptation that leads to the (wrong) action.

Fortunately, while cues are difficult to change, we can change the habits that follow them. If you currently have a cue that you absolutely have to eat something sugary at 2 PM, a craving will fire up in your brain exactly at 2 PM. The following habit – say, eating a piece of chocolate – is a guarantee unless you modify it.

If you give in and eat chocolate, you'll make the association stronger. If you resist – and replace it with a healthy alternative (say, an apple instead of a chocolate bar), given enough time you'll stop craving a chocolate bar and crave an apple instead. Granted, the first few tries will be difficult, but resisting the old action will get easier with time.

The tricky thing is to endure the period of change. It's easy to say "replace it with a healthy alternative." It's hard to do it when you can't stop thinking about a delicious chocolate cake.

There are several ways to beat your temptations. The first step is to…

Remove Temptations

Removing temptations from sight is the simplest and most effective strategy to deal with cravings.

If you don't have any forbidden foods at home, it will be easier to resist the temptation to cheat. If they're always within reach, you're making it unnecessarily hard for yourself to stick to your diet.

Start your commitment by emptying your fridge and pantry of unhealthy foods. Otherwise an unscheduled cheat day is bound to happen sooner than you think. This is not an optional piece of advice – it's mandatory if you're serious about your results.

There's a world of difference between a chocolate bar right there and 15 minutes away in a store.

In the first case, all you have to do is to take a few steps, open the fridge and there you go – the food is in your mouth. In the second case, you have to put on shoes, take the car keys, get in your car, drive to the store, find the food you're craving, buy it, and go back home. If a craving is weak, it's possible you won't be in the mood to do all of these things just to satisfy it.

The same advice applies to any other temptation-generating elements of the environment: TV (ads), driving nearby to your favorite fast food restaurants, etc.

If you have cravings at work and always go to a vending machine to grab something unhealthy, don't carry any money with you. It's possible you'll still be tempted to buy that candy bar, but what are you going to do without money? Borrow it from a colleague?

"Hey, George. Can you lend me five bucks so I can gorge on these delicious candy bars?" That should be enough of a deterrent not to do it.

If your daily routine includes driving by your favorite place, change the route so you won't be tempted to engage in your old habits.

If ads make you hungry, don't watch television, or leave the room during the ads. The fewer triggers that pester you on a daily basis, the easier it is to deal with cravings.

One time for a few days in a row, I was craving a particular chocolate bar. When I finally felt I could indulge, I wasn't in the mood to drive to the store just to buy it – and the craving was gone. I'm sure that if I had had it at home, I wouldn't have hesitated to eat it.

It's possible you're not aware of various cues that result in cravings. Making a list of situations in which you feel cravings the most will help you come up with ways to remove the temptations or dangerous cues. Let's say you write down:

- each time I drive past my favorite burger joint and want to stop and grab a bite,

- each time I pass the vending machine at work and realize it's lunch time,

- each time I don't eat a satisfying, tasty meal and feel the need to eat something flavorful,

- each time I have a nap and wake up with cravings for sugar,

- each time I meet with my friend for coffee and she orders a chocolate cake.

Now you can come up with ways to remove these situations and cues from your life. So:

- don't drive past your favorite burger joint. Find a different route, even if it requires a longer commute.

- don't walk past the vending machine if possible. If not, don't carry any cash and credit cards with you to work.

- learn how to cook tasty, filling meals or eat at a healthy restaurant. Do whatever you can to avoid bland meals and find tasty *and* healthy foods.

- stop taking naps if you can't control the cravings. If you can't live without naps, remove all types of sweets from your home (you should have done it by now, anyway) and leave only fruits. Soon, you'll develop a healthier habit to grab a piece after a nap.

- take your friend to another place where she can't order anything unhealthy. Eat a large, filling meal before meeting with her so you don't feel hungry. Carry only enough cash (and no credit card) to pay for coffee, and nothing else.

It's easier to remove the danger of a craving before you feel it than learn how to use your willpower to resist it. As they say, an ounce of prevention is worth a pound of cure. Make a plan of action and change your routines to improve your chances of success.

The Power of Waiting

In the famous Stanford experiment on delayed gratification, scientists offered children a choice between a small immediate reward (a marshmallow, a cookie, or a pretzel) or two small rewards 15 minutes later[xv]. During the waiting period the tester left the room, leaving children with the alluring reward at their fingertips. Some kids gave up and ate the reward right away, thus losing the two rewards later on, while others succeeded at resisting the temptation.

The subsequent follow-up studies have shown that the children who were able to resist the temptation were found to be more successful in life (as measured by SAT scores, incidence of behavioral problems and BMI)[xvi].

How did the kids deal with the temptation, especially when taking into account that children have little self-discipline when compared to adults? They distracted themselves.

As the leading researcher Walter Mischel observed, some would "cover their eyes with their hands or turn around so that they can't see the tray, others start kicking the desk, or tug on their pigtails, or stroke the marshmallow as if it were a tiny stuffed animal."

While it doesn't sound like a great strategy to stroke the chocolate bar you don't want to eat or kick your desk each time you're tempted to cave in, the idea behind it – self-distraction – is.

Waiting on the temptation for fifteen minutes is usually enough to reduce the craving or eliminate it altogether.

Whenever you feel a craving, tell yourself that you'll wait fifteen minutes, then make a decision whether you'll give in or not. If the craving is still there, give yourself another fifteen minutes.

While waiting for fifteen (or thirty, or sixty – whatever works for you) minutes before you take action to satisfy the craving, distract yourself. Better yet, instead of trying *not* to think about the temptation, try to focus on something else entirely until it passes.

Call your friend. Start watching a movie. Go for a walk. Play with your pet. Read something. Engage in a task you've been postponing for a long time (cleaning?). Whatever you choose, make sure you immerse yourself in the activity so you can get a respite from the craving.

Use Your Imagination to Kill Your Craving

Some types of unhealthy foods are so bad for you it's best to avoid them forever or eat them once in a blue moon. These include, among others: potato chips, soda (including diet soda with harmful artificial sweeteners), microwave popcorn (air-popped is fine), and sugary cereal.

How can you permanently destroy your cravings for these addictive foods if you've been eating them for a long time? You change your associations, which works almost like brainwashing yourself.

The technique is to make the food you crave as undesirable as possible. Instead of distracting yourself trying not to think about the craving, focus on the food you want to eat, but make it unappealing.

You can imagine stuffing your face with a chocolate bar and realize how unattractive and weak-minded you'll look. Remember how bloated or otherwise uncomfortable you feel after eating a certain unhealthy treat. Imagine eating it in front of an entire audience of people.

You can look up the ingredients of the food you want to eat and read about their negative effects on the body. Make it as real as possible. Read about the everyday life of extremely obese people, look up heart transplant in Wikipedia and imagine that could happen to you if you keep eating the food you crave.

Imagine lying in your death bed and your family members looking at you with sadness, everybody knowing that if it wasn't for your unhealthy diet, you would still be alive and kicking.

Think of the example you are setting for your children. Would you like them to be obese and unhealthy in the future because they had plenty of examples of you gorging on junk food?

Yes, I'm aware how distressing these examples are. It has to be uncomfortable and emotional to give you a boost of negative motivation. Ruin your positive associations with the food you crave and chances are you won't touch it (at least this time).

I used to eat crazy amounts of macaroni and cheese. It was one of my staple meals. I found it a challenge to stop eating it every single day, let alone permanently.

A few years of religiously following my new eating habits have fixed my dependence on mac and cheese, but I still sometimes crave it.

If I don't want to cheat on a given day when I feel the craving, I remind myself of how much it upsets my stomach. I try to imagine how quickly the taste goes from incredible (the first few bites) to merely okay (a few minutes later) to "I can't eat it any longer" (while there's still some food on the plate). I also remind myself of an uncomfortable picture of the stomach digesting pasta I once saw online.

As the hot-cold empathy gap says[xvii], we generally find it difficult to imagine and understand how it feels to be in an opposite state. If we're satiated, it's difficult to understand how hunger can take over our control. Or if we're angry or sad, it's difficult to understand how it feels to be happy. Or if we aren't sexually aroused, we fail to predict the kind of risky sexual decisions we can take while being in the "hot" state[xviii].

In the case of craving for mac and cheese, it's difficult to imagine that eating it will *not* be delicious. It's only when you give in that you can experience the emotion you would have never expected during your "hot" state (and then you find it hard to believe you couldn't have resisted the temptation given how unsatisfactory the experience turns out to be).

Being aware of this bias can help you avoid giving in to a temptation. Instead of (yet again) being puzzled as to why you imagined your forbidden food as so great (and finding out it's not really that incredible, and you only get guilt as a reward), think about it prior to making the wrong decision.

Imagine – as much as you can – that it won't taste as great as you think. Logic doesn't always work to avoid these wrong decisions (after all, it's an emotional craving), but it can help.

Use Your Progress to Fight Cravings

The most important reason why you should take measurements and pictures of your body is to track progress. If you don't know if you're slimming down or if your weight remains the same, it's difficult to maintain willpower and keep going.

There's another reason why you should do it, though – it's a powerful weapon when fighting cravings, especially in a later phase of dieting. If you take pictures every few weeks and weigh yourself on a weekly (or fortnightly) basis, it's easy to see progress and get a boost of motivation.

If you feel you're about to succumb to a craving, take a look at your progress photos and graphs of your weight going down. Ponder on the fact that if you give in, chances are you'll threaten your future progress. In many cases, it will be enough to resist the temptation or at least reduce its intensity.

Even when you complete your diet, it's a good habit to weigh yourself every week or so to control whether your new eating habits work for you or need to be changed. Don't rely on weight alone, though – measuring your waist and hips along with monitoring your weight gives a better picture of your physique. Such a simple tracking system will also help you maintain healthy habits and stave off cravings.

Schedule Your Cravings

It's useful to be a self-disciplined person, but it doesn't mean things have to be hard. The easier dieting is, the less likely you'll be to cave in to a temptation and give up.

In my case, by following a diet with a clearly designated weekly cheat day, I knew that I only had to postpone my cravings for a few days.

It wasn't required to give up my favorite unhealthy foods forever – it was just for a few days. After some time, I stopped craving these foods so much, so in the end taking the easy way out (cheating each week) was better than making things too challenging (not allowing myself any cheating).

Science also agrees that cheat meals are valuable. Overeating (while on a low-calorie diet) helps increase the production levels of leptin, a hormone-like protein that regulates body weight and energy, by nearly 30% for up to 24 hours[xix]. This post-cheating increase boosts metabolism and may also lead to improved motivation[xx].

The safest way to do a cheat day is to pick one specific day a week, let's say Saturday (due to the fact that most people eat socially during the weekends), and limit all of the unhealthy foods to that period of time from when you wake up to the moment you go to sleep.

When your flexible cheat day serves mostly as a physical break, eat whatever you want, how much you want (within reason – don't make yourself sick). The goal is to stop thinking about your diet, about any kinds of restrictions, and just enjoy food. One day of feasting won't ruin your entire progress (as long as you maintain a strict deficit during the remaining six days), and the psychological break will help adhere to a long term diet.

Keep just one thing in mind – no traces of your cheat day should remain in your fridge or in your pantry the next day. Eat everything you buy on the same day, or if you can't finish it, give it to someone else. Alternatively, give it to someone else for safekeeping until your next cheat day. Under no circumstances leave it at home – if you follow a cheat day with another unplanned cheat day, you'll most likely ruin your diet.

How to Get the Most Good Out of a Cheat Day

Unfortunately, only high-protein, high-carb, and low-fat cheat days affect the levels of leptin[xxi]. In other words, if your sole purpose of cheating is to boost your leptin levels, you have to say no to pizza, ice cream, chocolate, and other fatty foods.

Doesn't sound like a happy cheat day, does it? If you want to be strict about it, you can structure it this way. If you prefer flexibility at the expense of slower progress, don't control your cheat days so strictly.

There are both physiological and psychological effects of cheating. Even if you can't obtain the maximum physiological benefits because you choose not to have a low-fat day, you can still enjoy the psychological ones.

Giving yourself a scheduled break will save you guilt. Instead of entering the vicious post-guilt cycle ("I already screwed up, it doesn't make sense to get back on track") – which will surely happen, because few people can adhere to a strict diet with 100%

accuracy – you'll feel okay, knowing it was all planned beforehand.

It's about long-term commitment, not depriving yourself of everything and hoping you'll fight off every single temptation. As long as you maintain healthy eating habits 80-90% of time, you'll be fine. The longer you stick to a healthy diet, the better your health will become – even with occasional returns to less than healthy foods.

To reduce the negative effects of increased calorie consumption, consider beginning your cheat day with a glycogen-depleting workout on an empty stomach in the morning. A solid weightlifting session at the gym can do the trick.

Some people follow cheat days with fast days – days without eating anything at all or with just a small protein-rich meal. That's how I usually structure my cheat days – the day after increased calorie consumption is a day with zero calories, just water (tea and black coffee are allowed, too).

As bodybuilder and fitness coach John Romaniello writes, "giving your digestive system a day off has its benefits. Not only will it force your body to more efficiently utilize the caloric overload from the preceding cheat day, but you'll ALSO [sic] let the less than healthy stuff move out of your body a bit quicker"[xxii].

As long as you don't have any issues preventing you from having a fast day (speak with your doctor before trying it), it's a powerful way to supercharge your results when dieting – while also teaching you more self-control.

A fast day will not only let your digestive system recover, but also help you avoid any spillover effects from the cheat day. Moreover, it can increase your weight loss rate – after all, you get a deficit of your entire daily caloric consumption.

The day after a fast day eat what you normally eat during your regular day of dieting. Don't attempt to eat more calories to account for the previous day – the point is to skip them.If you feel that cheat days don't help you maintain long-term self-discipline, don't do them or do them less often. Depending on how strong-minded you feel when dieting, giving yourself a day off can remind you of the foods you'd like to stop eating and result in more cravings for the next week of dieting.

No matter what you decide regarding cheat days, avoid cheating on a daily basis. Eating small amounts of forbidden foods every day is worse than eating huge amounts of forbidden foods once a week.

In the first case, it does nothing to help you break the habit of eating unhealthy. You'll still be used to the taste of the unhealthy foods and look forward to them every day. In the second case, you'll eat them less often, so you'll have more time to disaccustom yourself and permanently change your eating habits.

What to Do When You Give In

As effective as the techniques I've shared with you are, it's almost a guarantee you won't always resist the temptation. If you succumb to a craving or have an unscheduled cheat day, the risk of failure soars. However, it's not the act of eating forbidden foods in itself that will ruin your diet, but your psychological response.

People who experience a failure when dieting can react in two ways:

1. Despair, call themselves weak-minded and victimize themselves. There's only one outcome for this behavior – diet failure. A few weeks or months later they start again, only to fail again when they beat themselves up again after another little failure.

2. Acknowledge the mistake, try to identify what has made them slip up, remind themselves that they're not perfect but it's all about the process and move on. Success is guaranteed for these people.

If you slip up, don't beat yourself up. More often than not, self-guilt will only exacerbate the problem. Instead of thinking "I slipped up, but now I'll get back on track," guilt will make you think "I'm a failure. It makes no sense to follow the diet any longer."

Acknowledge you've made a mistake and move on. One slip-up won't ruin your progress unless you let it by feeling overly guilty about it. It's about the long-term process, and not just one event.

HOW TO DEAL WITH CRAVINGS: QUICK RECAP

1. Cues trigger cravings. It's hard to change a cue, but it's possible to change the subsequent routine (like eating a piece of chocolate). The key is to repeatedly – without a fault – keep performing the new action instead of the old one for as long as needed to establish a new habit, generally at least 66 days.

2. The simplest way to endure cravings is to remove temptations from your surroundings. The more difficult it is to satisfy your cravings, the less likely you'll be to act on them.

Compare having a piece of chocolate within your reach and the necessity to drive to the store to buy it. If you're tired after work, it's possible your laziness will win over the craving.

Make a list of all the situations and signals that make you feel cravings and find reasonable ways to remove them from your life, or at least greatly reduce the risk you won't be able to overcome the temptation (for instance, by eating a filling meal before meeting with a friend in a fast food restaurant).

3. Waiting for the craving to pass is the simplest, and probably the most effective way to deal with it. The trick is to distract yourself (or shift your focus) for long enough to let the feeling pass. Ideally, don't obsess about *not* thinking about the craving, but find something else to do that will shift your focus.

4. You can kill cravings by imagining in great detail bad things that will happen if you eat a particular unhealthy food. You can research what it's doing to your body over the long term. You can imagine yourself succumbing to a craving, failing with your diet, and becoming morbidly obese. Make it emotional and vivid, and it's possible the craving will pass.

Bear in mind that due to the hot-cold empathy gap, we're bad at predicting how we will feel in a "hot" state if we're currently in a "cold" state (and vice versa). For this reason, don't expect to possess the same level of self-control you have when hungry as when your stomach is full. Likewise, don't expect the food you crave to taste as incredible when eating (in the "cold" state) as when you imagine it while craving it (the "hot" state).

5. Take regular measurements and pictures of your body. Whenever you feel a craving, see them to remind yourself how far you've already come and that you don't want to ruin it by succumbing to a temptation.

6. In the beginning stages of dieting, cravings rarely go away. If you know you'll be able to satisfy them in just a few days (by scheduling cheat days), it will be easier to handle them. All you have to do is postpone them. Weekly cheat days offer a valuable psychological respite as well as offer other benefits for your body that can help boost your weight loss rate. For maximum benefits, consider beginning your cheat day with a workout and following it with a fast day (just don't follow it with another cheat day).

7. Don't feel guilty when you slip up. Acknowledge your mistake, learn your lesson, and move on. If you spend too much time thinking about

it, guilt-motivated eating can send you into a downward spiral.

Chapter 3: How to Part Ways with Unhealthy Food

It's a long and exhausting battle to fight unhealthy foods and come out victorious. Temptations – the little soldiers unhealthy foods use to lure you into a trap – are everywhere. Even if somebody locked you up in a room surrounded by piles of vegetables and fruits for weeks, the moment you got out you'd be running to the nearest store or restaurant for something unhealthy.

Consequently, we need to learn how to come up with healthy and tasty alternatives for unhealthy foods (so you don't postpone your cravings, but replace them altogether), learn how to improve the taste of healthy foods (they need more work than your typical junk food), and handle restrictions the right way. And these are precisely the type of concepts we'll cover in this chapter.

Come up with Healthy and Tasty Alternatives

As I've already noted in my previous book, *Daily Self-Discipline*, missing their favorite foods like pizza, chocolate, ice cream, or french fries isn't the only reason people can't overcome cravings. They also cave in because they never develop permanent alternatives to them. Here are some of the tips I gave in the previous book with some additional advice...

Unless you develop an enjoyable alternative to the unhealthy foods you love, you'll always miss them so much that resisting cravings will be very difficult.

If there's no healthy food that can give you at least half of the enjoyment of the unhealthy food, sooner or later you won't resist the temptation to eat it. In an ideal world, you would. In the real world, willpower can rarely last so long.

However, can you guess how easy it is to maintain a diet that lets you eat all that you want? The key is to find healthy alternatives that give you what you want (that normally comes from unhealthy foods).

There are usually certain things we miss from a particular unhealthy food. If it's chocolate, maybe you miss the sweet flavor. Maybe it's the texture and the sweet flavor. Maybe it's just the smell. If you crave pizza, maybe what you crave the most is melted cheese. If you can figure out what you miss the most, it will be easier to come up with alternatives.

Let's be honest here – you can't replace the perfect, sweet taste of chocolate melting on your tongue with a stalk of bland broccoli. However, you can probably do it (to some extent – enough to not miss chocolate every single day) with:

- all kinds of berries (strawberries, raspberries, blueberries – is there anyone who doesn't love them?),

- dark chocolate (it's much healthier, and due to its deep taste – we're talking about 70% cacao content here – you need much less to satisfy your sweet tooth),

- smoothies (just don't go overboard with them – that's a lot of fructose),

- high-quality honey (there's a world of difference between cheap store honey and homemade organic varieties – experiment with various flavors)

- carob (while not entirely something you can eat on a daily basis as a healthy alternative, it's better than regular chocolate)

How about pizza? You can learn how to do it yourself with whole-wheat flour, homemade tomato sauce, organic vegetables, and high-quality cheese. You can also cook a frittata or quiche, both of which can imitate pizza pretty well.

Ice cream? You can eat natural frozen yogurt and mix in some berries instead of eating store-bought ice cream. You can also make it yourself. If you opt for regular ice cream, at least buy ice cream with as few ingredients as possible (e.g. plain vanilla or strawberry ice cream).

French fries? Either learn how to make them at home and use healthy oils to fry them or learn how to cook baked potatoes. There are also various alternatives with other vegetables – seasoned pepper sticks, carrot fries, baked zucchini chips, or kale chips.

Improve the Taste of Healthier Foods

Spices and herbs have a lot to do with taste. Many vegetables rarely taste good alone. However, if you add the right spice or herb to them, they get much tastier – oftentimes so tasty, you develop a craving for these foods. To give you a few examples, here are spices and/or herbs that dramatically change the taste of certain healthy foods:

1. Eggs: chives, salt, and/or black pepper. Scrambled eggs alone can be a bit bland. Adding any of these makes the taste much better. If you don't enjoy eating eggs alone, eat them as a sandwich with a slice of whole wheat bread and cheese. Just keep in mind it won't be as satiating as a meal in which grains are replaced with an additional serving of vegetables.

2. Zucchini: cayenne pepper, basil, cumin, garlic powder, oregano, or thyme. A lot of herbs and spices go well with zucchini. Few people enjoy this

vegetable alone, but adding just a pinch or two of any of these flavor-intensifiers can make a world of difference – especially if you grill it. This applies to many other vegetables, too – for instance, eggplant, squash, or pumpkin.

3. Brown rice: turmeric, cumin, or soy sauce. Most people used to eating white rice are not as happy with the taste of brown rice. Try combining it with turmeric or cumin or add soy sauce. You can also check Asian spice mixes for rice. Don't forget you don't have to stick to regular brown rice. Wild rice or black rice are healthy alternatives to white rice, too. You can also try rice alternatives like quinoa, which, by the way, is a perfect pseudo-grain for vegetarians due to being a complete protein.

4. Vegetable soups: salt, black pepper, allspice, bay leaf, and/or garden lovage. Also, add a lot of onions to improve the flavor. Simple everyday vegetable soups are perfect for anyone who doesn't like cooking every single day. You can make a big pot of soup on Monday and eat it until Thursday.

With the right mix of spices, you can certainly develop a craving for soup (like I have).

5. Potatoes: salt, rosemary, paprika, oregano, basil, cayenne pepper, dill, and/or parsley. Potatoes, when eaten in moderation and not in the form of french fries, aren't as unhealthy as people believe. The key is to avoid frying them, instead opting for healthier methods, ideally by steaming. Once you come up with your perfect mix of herbs and spices, steamed potatoes might become more appealing than oil-coated french fries.

The way in which you cook vegetables (or other healthy foods) also makes a world of difference. Boiled potatoes taste different than baked potatoes. Steamed zucchini might have a horrible taste for you, but you could find baked zucchini chips addictive. Brown rice alone can be bland, but mixing it with beans can make it one of your staple meals.

You don't have to be a perfect cook to try different ways of preparing healthy foods. You're unlikely to mess something up when following basic recipes like baked potatoes, zucchini chips, or steaming vegetables. And even if you mess it up, next time will be better.

Mixing certain vegetables instead of eating them alone can also make a difference. Consider making a salad – you probably won't eat iceberg lettuce or red cabbage alone. However, when you mix them with carrots, bell peppers, eggs, grated parmesan, and olive oil, you can have a fulfilling, flavorful meal.

Experimentation can go a long way to avoid, or at least greatly reduce cravings for certain foods. Once you develop permanent alternatives you find as tasty (or tastier) than what you have craved, maintaining your healthy eating habits will get easier.

If you have no idea how to replace certain unhealthy foods with healthier alternatives, type "healthy alternatives to [unhealthy food you crave]" in Google. While not all alternatives will be as tasty as what you crave, perhaps with some tweaking they'll give you some ideas how to create a perfect replacement meal to curb your cravings.

Approach this exercise with an open mind. Some healthy alternatives will be ridiculous (e.g., replacing pasta with "Beetroot Ravioli" – one of the recipes I've found when searching for alternatives to pasta). Most won't taste as great as what you crave. But that will be your starting point.

I'd be the last person to say that healthy foods are tastier than the unhealthy ones. In the beginning stages of dieting, when you're still used to different, more addictive flavors, healthy foods are poor substitutes for the explosive flavor of pizza or the sweet taste of soda. However, trying different foods and getting used to different, more subtle flavors will sooner or later modify your taste buds to enjoy things you've never liked before. It's like re-training your body to enjoy what's good for it.

For a long time I wouldn't touch broccoli or cauliflower. They smelled bad and tasted even worse. For that matter, most vegetables didn't look, smell, or taste particularly enticing. It was only when I started experimenting and learned how to spice them properly that I developed an affinity for them.

Today when I see a plate of steamed vegetables I think of it as a tasty meal, and not as a punishment for trying to be a healthy person (you won't go far with this mindset). If you keep exploring new tastes, sooner or later you'll find healthy foods that won't require willpower just to eat them.

Have a Food Journal

The participants of a study on weight loss from Kaiser Permanente's Center for Health Research who kept diet records lost twice as much weight as those who kept no records[xxiii].

There was nothing magical about their journals – as Keith Bachman, MD, a Kaiser Permanente internist and weight management specialist says, "Keeping a food diary doesn't have to be a formal thing. Just the act of scribbling down what you eat on a Post-It note, sending yourself e-mails tallying each meal, or sending yourself a text message will suffice. It's the process of reflecting on what we eat that helps us become aware of our habits, and hopefully change our behavior."

This practice can also help you develop more self-awareness, and consequently improve your self-discipline when on a diet. Eating a pizza is one thing.

Making yourself painfully aware of it by noting it down in your food journal makes it "more real" – suddenly it's there as proof of your wrong choice.

If you can combine it with the power of being held accountable – say, showing your food journal to your (demanding) family member weekly – staying away from unhealthy food will be easier.

Go Easy on Restrictions

Dieting is not a sprint – it's a marathon. If you have more than 20 pounds to lose, it will take you months to reach your perfect weight. As long as you don't have any pressing health concerns that require you to lose weight *right now*, you don't have to start your diet with overly restrictive rules.

Designating one day per week as a cheat day is a good way to go easy on restrictions, because you don't have to go cold turkey with unhealthy food. You just postpone eating these foods for a few days, and then you can partake again.

Later on, if you no longer feel you require weekly cheat days, you can turn them into a fortnightly thing. Or you can designate cheat meals, not entire cheat days. The idea is to start from something easy – being able to cheat weekly – and gradually eat unhealthy food less and less often.

Another simple way to go easy on restrictions is to start your diet by making a small, almost unnoticeable change in your diet.

For instance, on day one you replace one type of unhealthy food with something healthier (e.g., blueberries instead of a chocolate bar). Then you maintain it for as long as needed until it feels natural and you feel you can handle more restrictions.

Then you can reduce your portions of unhealthy foods by 10% (and increasing your portions of healthy foods by 10%) – another small change that, given enough time, will become another of your unnoticeable routines on your way toward more health.

A week or two later (or however long you need to feel ready to move on), make yet another change – for instance, stop eating an entire group of unhealthy foods (e.g. processed meats) during the week and let yourself eat it only on your designated cheat day.

such a slow, gradual approach will be
your willpower and thus make it easier to
part ways with unhealthy foods.

Wean Off the Most Addictive Foods

A 2015 study on addictive foods conducted by the scientists at the University Michigan and the New York Obesity Research Center shows that the 10 most addictive foods are[xxiv]:

1. Pizza – a mean rating of 4.01, with 1 being the easiest to resist and 7 being the most difficult to resist

2. Chocolate – 3.73 (tie)

3. Chips – 3.73 (tie)

4. Cookies – 3.71

5. Ice cream – 3.68

6. French fries – 3.60

7. Cheeseburgers – 3.51

8. Soda (not diet) – 3.29

9. Cake – 3.26

10. Cheese – 3.22

Unsurprisingly, all of these foods (perhaps with the exception of cheese) are unhealthy and make you hungry again quickly after you eat them. If you want to change the proportions and eat healthy food 80-90% of the time (including cheat days), start eliminating the foods from the top of the list first as these are the ones that deplete your willpower the most.

Slowly transition to less addictive foods and/or rotate them, so that even if you allow yourself to cheat weekly, you won't eat the most addictive foods regularly.

If, for instance, you eat pizza every cheat day, eat it every two weeks and slowly replace it with something less addictive. You can eat whole wheat pizza or make it yourself to make it healthier and less addictive. You can also rotate it with french fries, a cheeseburger, or ice cream to eat it only once a month.

The less often you eat it, the weaker your addiction to it will become. Then it will be easier to resist it, and you'll clean up your eating habits permanently.

Speaking of addictive foods, be particularly cautious about "I'll eat only a little bit of it" foods –

foods that you can't stop eating after just a "little bit" as you promise yourself. One example is peanut butter. Few people who like peanut butter can eat just a spoonful of it and be done.

The same applies to other, usually fat-rich or carb-rich foods, that cast a spell on you the moment you eat just a small amount (popcorn would be another example here – very few eat just a handful).

HOW TO PART WAYS WITH UNHEALTHY FOOD: QUICK RECAP

1. If you don't come up with healthy, tasty alternatives to the unhealthy foods you crave, you'll never be able to part ways with them. Dieting is easier when you have several go-to healthy meals you're looking forward to (vs dreading them).

2. Consider what you miss from a particular unhealthy food and come up with foods that can mimic or give you what you crave. For instance, if you want to eat chocolate, perhaps you crave something sweet. In this case, berries, honey, or 70%+ dark chocolate can do the trick.

3. Spices and herbs can make a dramatic difference to healthy foods that usually have a bland taste. Even a simple addition of salt and pepper is enough to transform a previously unpalatable food into something you're looking forward to eating.

4. Experiment with various ways of cooking healthy foods. Boiled vegetables have a different taste than fried vegetables, which have a different flavor than baked vegetables.

5. Keep a food journal to become more aware of what you put in your body. If you can, find someone who will keep you accountable by browsing through your food journal each week.

6. Go easy on restrictions. It's not necessary to quit cold turkey and stop eating all types of unhealthy foods forever. Even if it takes you months before you eliminate most of the unhealthy foods from your daily menu, it's still a step in the right direction.

7. Highly-processed foods are the most addictive foods. If you want to part ways with unhealthy food, start with eliminating these foods first. If you're already on a diet and have weekly cheat days, try not to eat the same addictive food each week. Rotate it with other treats to wean off it.

Chapter 4: Scientifically-Based Tricks to Improve Satiety

There are two approaches you can use to better stick to your diet:

First, you can use various psychological tricks to motivate yourself to keep going – create negative associations with your cravings, schedule your cravings for a cheat day later during the week, or distract yourself with something else.

The other approach explored in this chapter is to use simple, scientifically-based tricks to improve satiety and consequently make willpower less relevant.

Eat More Dietary Fiber

Many nutrition experts recommend eating foods high in fiber for increased satiety and reduced calorie intake. However, the reality is different, and while the advice is partially true, you can't eat any kind of fiber to enjoy these benefits.

According to a 2013 meta-analysis on the effect of fiber on satiety and food intake, out of the 38 fiber types studied for satiety effects, only beta-glucan, lupin kernel fiber, rye bran, whole grain rye, or a mixed high-fiber diet were supported in more than one publication as satiety-enhancing[xxv]. Some other types of fiber were supported in one publication, which from the scientific point of view isn't enough proof that they're indeed effective.

Consequently, there are only a few types of food rich in fiber that will enhance your satiety. These include:

- containing beta-glucan: oats and barley. Beta-glucan is also found in mushrooms like reishi, shiitake, chaga and maitake[xxvi].

- containing lupin kernel fiber: lupin beans.

- rye bran, whole rye bread, and similar foods.

If you're going to eat bread while dieting, opt for whole rye, oat, or barley bread. When compared to regular white bread, these foods will be more satiating and possibly reduce your overall calorie intake.

Keep in mind it doesn't mean that it's not worth it to eat other foods rich in dietary fiber. Fiber provides more benefits than just increased satiety. Vegetables should still be a staple of your diet. The aforementioned sources of fiber can support you while dieting, especially when you want to keep eating grains while on a diet.

Eat More Protein

Protein is more satiating than fats or carbohydrates[xxvii]. If you eat a high-protein diet, you'll feel hunger less often than a person who eats less of it. It will also help you lose more fat mass.

A Danish study has shown that a group following a fat-reduced diet (30% of energy) high in protein (25% of energy) for 6 months achieved a substantially greater weight loss (9.4 vs 5.9 kg, or 20.8 lbs vs 13 lbs) than a group following the same fat-reduced diet medium in protein (12% of energy)[xxviii].

After 12 months, the weight loss of the high-protein group wasn't significantly higher than the medium-protein group (6.2 and 4.3 kg, or 13.6 lbs and 9.5 lbs), but it had a 10% greater reduction in intra-abdominal adipose tissue (in layman's terms, your stomach fat).

A 2008 paper "Protein, Weight Management, and Satiety" concludes that "a moderate increase in dietary protein in association with physical activity and an energy-controlled diet may improve the regulation of body weight by ... increasing satiety"[xxix].

Satiety is the key word here. As Australian professor Manny Noakes at the Commonwealth Scientific and Industrial Research Organisation writes in her 2008 paper, "Studies comparing ad libitum high protein diets to high carbohydrate diets have usually shown greater weight loss on the high protein pattern and that enhanced satiety was the most important factor in the weight loss"[xxx].

Okay, enough studies. How can you apply it to your diet? It's simple – increase the amount of protein in your diet. You'll be less likely to suffer from hunger. Consequently, you'll eat less and lose weight more quickly with less problems.

You don't necessarily need to count every single gram of protein in your diet. Just make sure you eat at least one protein-rich food with each meal so you get roughly 30-40 grams of protein per meal. If you prefer counting, 2.3-3.1 g per kg (~1.1-1.4 g per lb) of lean body mass[xxxi] is the amount of protein you should consume when dieting.

Foods high in protein include:

- meat – opt for lean meat like chicken or turkey. Avoid processed meats (sausages, hot dogs, canned meat).

- fish – choose wild fish over farmed.

- eggs – considered the perfect protein. Go for free-range and cage-free sources.

- dairy – good choices include cottage cheese, Greek yogurt, high-quality Swiss cheese and 2% or full milk.

- quinoa – a vegetarian source of all of the essential amino acids.

- legumes – usually combined with rice to form a complete, strong protein.

In general, animal sources of protein are better than plant sources because animal sources contain all essential amino acids. Most plant sources don't have all of them, so you have to combine various sources to get all the amino acids your body needs.

While it's possible to increase your protein intake with supplements (whey protein being the most common choice), it's always better to opt for whole foods. They're more satiating than a shake, and taste better, too.

If you find it hard to eat enough protein, don't like to cook much, don't have time to cook, or simply want to supplement your intake with supplements, go with whey protein. Real food is always better than supplements, but whey protein can be a worthy addition to your diet – and not only if you're a bodybuilder.

According to a 2013 review by Japanese scientists Rie Tsutsumi and Yasuo M. Tsutsumi, peptides and proteins found in whey protein are likely to result in beneficial changes for both healthy and diseased individuals[xxxii].

Some of the potential beneficial effects of whey protein include: reduced fasting insulin levels in the obese and overweight[xxxiii], increased satiety when compared with casein (cheese is made mostly of casein)[xxxiv], reduced food intake when consumed as a whey-enriched yoghurt drink[xxxv], and resting energy expenditure when consumed before sleep[xxxvi].

Please keep in mind that while all of these benefits sound incredible, you can enjoy the same – if not better benefits – by simply sticking to a high-protein diet of real, unprocessed foods. Whey protein is not necessary for optimal health, but can help if you otherwise find it hard to consume enough protein.

Choose the Most Satiating Foods and Go for Volume

A 1995 study conducted by Suzanna Holt and her fellow researchers at the University of Sydney on a satiety index of common foods has shown that the foods that weigh the most are best at satisfying hunger (regardless of the number of calories they contain). High content of protein, fiber, and water were correlated with increased satiety, while fat content and palatability were negatively associated with it.

The difference in satiety among 38 studied foods was astounding. Boiled potatoes (with the highest Satiety Index score) were seven times more satiating than a croissant (with the lowest Satiety Index score).

Based partly on these findings, the leading site with nutrition data, NutritionData.Self.com, created a mathematical formula that predicts satiety from the nutrient content of a given food or recipe[xxxvii].

The resulting Fullness Factor, falling within the range of 0 to 5 (with foods with high FF's being more satiating), makes it easy to find foods that are best at satiating your hunger, and thus reducing your hunger and helping you stick to a diet better.

Some of the common foods highest in Fullness Factor include:

- bean sprouts,

- watermelon,

- grapefruit,

- carrots,

- oranges.

Some of the common foods lowest in Fullness Factor include:

- butter,

- potato chips,

- honey,

- white bread,

- ice cream.

If you're looking for the most satiating foods in a particular food group, you can refer to NutritionData.Self.com. Head over to their Nutritional Target Map Search and click the top right area of the graph (so it shows Fullness Factor and ND Rating of 5.0). The resulting foods will be the most satiating and most nutritionally dense.

Unsurprisingly, the most satiating foods are vegetables and some fruits. If you go for volume with these foods, you won't find yourself as hungry as with other choices.

If you want to feel the difference, eat a pound (~0.5 kg) of broccoli (use spices to make them tastier). Fullness Factor for broccoli is 4.2, and a pound of broccoli amounts to about 175 calories (that's about 5-15% of daily caloric intake for a person on a diet). Note down how hungry you feel two hours after eating this meal.

Then compare it to about two slices of toasted white bread with a Fullness Factor of 1.9. Two slices – that weigh about two ounces (50 grams) – contain about the same amount of calories as a pound of broccoli, which is ten times more in volume. You probably won't even have to wait two hours to feel hungry again after eating such an unsatisfactory meal – most likely you'll still be hungry right after the meal.

Another benefit of filling foods is that it's very difficult to overeat them. You can't consume a thousand worth of calories in, say, raw carrots in one sitting – that would require eating over five pounds (or 2.5 kg) of them. Now compare it to a small, 8-ounce (230 grams) bag of potato chips that has 1,242 calories.

That's the powerful difference when making vegetables the staple of your diet in comparison to sticking to your old, unhealthy eating habits that can't even keep you full for thirty minutes.

Prepare meals consisting of foods high in Fullness Factor and your diet will require much less willpower to maintain. Ideally, come up with several staple filling meals you can cook in less than 15 minutes, and if you find yourself hungry, snack on them.

SCIENTIFICALLY-BASED TRICKS TO STICK TO A DIET: QUICK RECAP

1. There are a few types of food rich in dietary fiber that are proven to increase satiety and consequently reduce the amount of calories you need to consume to feel full. They include: oats, barley, whole rye bread, lupin beans, and mushrooms like reishi, shiitake, chaga, and maitake.

2. Protein is more satiating than fats or carbohydrates. It helps achieve more fat loss, and particularly burn more belly fat. Try to eat roughly 30-40 grams of protein per meal, or 2.3-3.1 g per kg (~1.1-1.4 g per lb) of lean body mass a day to benefit from the beneficial effects of protein.

3. Foods high in protein include meat, fish, eggs, dairy, quinoa, and legumes. Animal sources of protein are more beneficial because they contain all essential amino acids your body needs to function properly. Whey protein can be a valuable addition to your diet if you can't otherwise provide your body with enough protein.

4. Not all foods are equal satiety-wise. Use the Fullness Factor to find the most satiating foods and make them the basis of your diet. In general, foods that satiate the most are vegetables (including kale, broccoli, cauliflower, etc.) and some kinds of fruits like watermelons and oranges. Highly processed foods usually have little effect on satiety, and they leave you as hungry as before you ate them.

Chapter 5: Most Common Willpower-Related Problems and Excuses When Dieting

Dieting comes with a lot of challenges, and while some of them are legitimate, many are excuses in disguise. In this chapter, we'll cover some of the most common problems when dieting which are actually just convenient rationalizations for sticking to unhealthy foods.

Once you get to know the solutions to these problems, you'll no longer be able to make excuses as doing so would only uncover that it's not a legitimate problem, but just a lack of self-discipline on your part.

I Eat Unhealthy Food Because I Don't Have Time

Underlying problem: you don't have enough self-discipline to come up with time-efficient ways to prepare healthy foods (and change your routine so you introduce these ideas in your life).

Out of all the excuses for eating unhealthy food, this one is one of the most notorious, and also one of the easiest to deal with. Here's how you can solve this problem:

1. Stock up on frozen foods

According to the study led by Ronald B. Pegg at the Department of Food Science & Technology at the University of Georgia, frozen veggies are similar to, and sometimes better, than fresh ones. As the scientists note, "This makes sense, considering that these veggies are usually flash-frozen (which suspends/pauses their 'aging' and nutrient losses) immediately after being harvested. Frozen veggies are often picked in the peak of their season, too"[xxxviii].

Frozen foods don't take much time to prepare. In fact, in many cases, all you need to do is to steam them for fifteen minutes and they're ready to go — often as a perfect meal that doesn't require any adjustments besides spicing it.

How much willpower do you need to buy a few bags of frozen food and put them in your steamer? It doesn't involve cleaning, slicing, or thinking which vegetables to mix – it's all ready for you.

2. Cook meals that you can store for a few days.

My favorite suggestion here is soups. True, it takes some time to prepare them if you need to clean and slice all of the vegetables, but if you make a large pot it will last you a good 3-4 days. Reheating soup doesn't require anything from you besides an occasional stir.

Other foods that can be stored for a few days and still taste great include frittatas, chili, roasted veggies, and salads.

Will it really be that time-consuming to spend an hour to cook enough food to last you three or four dinners?

3. Get someone else to cook for you.

If you can afford it, consider ordering your food from a healthy meal delivery service.

There are more and more companies that cook healthy meals and deliver them straight to your door. Most of them offer a few different menus to choose from; including vegetarian, paleo, and low-carb options.

While it's definitely more expensive to order food from such a service than cook it yourself, it can save you a lot of time you can invest into something else that will turn out more profitable in the end (e.g. growing your company or putting in more work to get a promotion).

Healthy restaurants are also an option, though these don't necessarily save a lot of time. After all, you have to leave your house and wait until they cook the food for you.

Don't forget there are more options to get someone else to cook for you than just these two. If you have a roommate who enjoys cooking, you can pay him or her to cook an additional meal for you. If you can afford it, you can also hire a part-time cook for you (though perhaps not a world-class chef, but simply a person who enjoys cooking and is looking for a way to make some money on the side, e.g. a retiree).

4. Realize that if you don't make time for health, you'll have to make time for illness.

If you have an unhealthy diet, it's not a question of "if" you get sick – it's "when." Hypertension, diabetes, heart disease, high cholesterol levels, cancer, ulcers, back pain, gallstones – these are just a few disorders and diseases an obese person will sooner or later develop.

If you value your time so much, it makes more sense to develop healthy (and time-efficient) habits to protect yourself from these problems. In the end, both the monetary and the time cost of health disorders and diseases will be much higher than prevention.

I Can't Afford Healthy Food

Underlying problem: you don't have enough self-discipline to learn which healthy foods are cheap, what you can do with them to prepare tasty meals, and how to calculate long-term costs of "saving" on healthy foods.

Healthy foods can be cheaper than junk food. For instance, most vegetables and fruits cost pennies when compared to highly processed foods. If you buy them from a local farmers market, it's even cheaper.

According to a 2013 meta-analysis by the scientists at the Harvard School of Public Health a day's worth of the healthiest foods cost about $1.50 more per day than the least healthy ones[xxxix].

That's about $550 per year more, but let's not forget about the costs of *not* eating healthy foods. Common medications can quickly add up to more than $550 per year, and much more if you suffer from lingering health disorders. Then there are increasing insurance costs, the costs of visiting a doctor (time, fuel), etc. Is it still worth it to "save money" on unhealthy foods?

You don't necessarily have to buy everything organic – vegetables are still vegetables, and it's better to eat non-organic veggies than not eat them at all. When scientists study the beneficial effects of vegetables and foods, they usually study conventional vegetables – not the organic ones – so don't worry about not getting the healthy benefits of eating vegetables if you can't afford the organic ones.

Healthy foods are usually more filling than the unhealthy ones. As we've already covered in the last chapter, you would need to eat over five pounds of broccoli to provide the same amount of calories as from a small bag of potato chips. However, a pack of chips wouldn't satisfy you at all, while even just a half of a pound of broccoli can be enough to fill you.

Consequently, vegetables and fruits that usually cost a dollar or less will provide a more satisfying and filling meal in the end – while paying either a bit more, the same, or less money than when ordering food from a dollar menu in a fast food restaurant.

Healthy Food Tastes Bad

Underlying problem: you don't have enough self-discipline to do a few experiments in the kitchen and create staple, tasty healthy meals.

Some healthy foods indeed do taste bad. But to say that all of them aren't flavorful is just an excuse to rationalize why you keep eating junk food.

It doesn't take much energy and time to come up with a few staple meals so you can always have something tasty to fall back on whenever you're hungry. These simple types of foods can include soups, potato- and vegetable-based recipes (e.g., boiled potatoes with some broccoli and fried eggs), rice and beans, or omelets and other egg-based meals.

As we've already covered in Chapter 3, spices and herbs make a lot of difference to the flavor of many healthy meals. Even using the right amount of salt and pepper alone can make a bland food flavorful. All you need is a modicum of willpower to cook a few meals and learn how to season them for perfect taste.

When I tried cooking a vegetable soup for the first time, it was as bland as it could get. It was unpalatable. However, it turned out I didn't use enough salt, pepper and other spices. Each time I tried it again, I improved my spice mix. Today, my vegetable soup – a staple in my diet I usually cook to keep for three days – is delicious, with the ideal flavor-enriching combination of spices and herbs.

If you don't get discouraged after your first tries, you'll develop your own recipes that will be both healthy and tasty. And your guests will love them as well.

If you find it challenging to cook or can never get the seasoning right, buy ready spice mixes. For instance, you can buy roasted or mashed potato seasoning mix, or get a mix of spices ready to use in a vegetable soup. Some frozen foods come with spice mixes, so you can't have it easier – just steam the vegetables and season them with what the manufacturer provided (make sure the mix doesn't contain any unhealthy flavor intensifiers like MSG).

Last but not least, many healthy foods are delicious without any additions. These include apples, bananas, berries, Greek yogurt, nuts, or melon. High-quality cheese, oatmeal, and eggs can also make healthy and tasty meals without a lot of cooking time or a need to add many seasonings.

I'm Hungry on a Diet

Underlying problem: you stick to unsatisfying foods or can't deal with the cravings for unhealthy foods.

If you're constantly hungry on a weight loss diet, there's something wrong with it. While you can't avoid an occasional feeling of hunger when you provide your body with fewer calories than your body needs, following a few simple rules can make this problem a non-issue:

1. Always start your meals with a portion of protein, the most satiating nutrient. Protein-rich foods include meat, fish, eggs, dairy, beans, and quinoa.

2. Each meal should come with a serving of vegetables (ideally) or fruits. Vegetables (along with some fruits) are the most filling foods.

3. Drink enough water. It's possible you mistake hunger with thirst. Whenever you feel hunger pangs, drink a cup of water. If they pass, you need to drink more water, not get more calories.

The feeling of hunger can also be related to eating bland, unsatisfying foods. While they can fill your stomach, oftentimes you still feel hungry after the meal due to their weak flavor – you're hungry for a specific taste. Make sure your meals satisfy your taste buds while still being good for you.

Another possible reason for being hungry on a diet is when your deficit is too high. Usually it doesn't make sense to create a long-term deficit higher than 500 calories or so a day (3500 kcal a week) as the increased difficulty of resisting temptations can lead to a diet failure instead of helping you lose weight more quickly.

What's the Point if I Gain Back the Weight Anyway?

Underlying problem: the wrong attitude.

If you start your diet thinking that you'll fail, then there's no point in dieting – you'll definitely gain back the weight, and probably even more than you had before.

A positive attitude and self-belief are one of the keys for success. Until you fix your attitude and start believing you can make permanent changes in your life, it's a waste of time to try to lose weight.

Developing a positive mindset starts with building confidence in your ability to change. If you've never had much luck with making permanent changes in your life, start with something small.

Consider introducing little habits in your life and repeating them until they become an inherent part of your life. Even such a little habit as daily flossing can help you build more belief in yourself and your ability to change.

Once you have some self-change experience under your belt, going on a diet or changing some of your eating habits will be less challenging. You'll have some lessons to draw out of your previous successful attempts at change and that will help your resolve.

Self-discipline is like a muscle. If you've never been to the gym and a coach tells you to lift 300 pounds off the ground, you won't be able to do it. But if he tells you to start with 50 pounds and increase the poundage weekly, sooner or later you will be exercising with 300 pounds.

Dieting is the same. If you have little willpower and little experience with introducing new habits, you don't necessarily have to begin with a full-blown diet. Start with a habit of eating a serving of vegetables a day. Feel your willpower strengthen. Then add another habit – e.g., limit sweets to three times a week.

When you feel your self-discipline can withstand more restrictions and you start believing in your ability to make permanent changes, consider starting a proper diet.

I Deserve a Treat

Underlying problem: small instant rewards mean more to you than postponed, but more valuable ones.

I know it's tempting to grab something sweet after a hard day. An hour-long walk makes you feel you deserve to reward yourself for the effort. It feels good to sit in front of the TV with potato chips or microwaved popcorn and a can of soda.

In all of these cases, it's like taking one step forward and two steps back. You burn 200 calories on your walk and consume 500 as a reward. You resist temptations for the entire day and then go crazy in the evening.

Treats can work given that they're limited to cheat days and serve as an infrequent respite. However, if you consistently reward yourself with something that sets you back, it's nothing else but a sure-fire way to fail.

There are two problems to solve here. Firstly, it's robbing your future self for the benefit of your present self. Most likely, you do it because you find it hard to imagine consequences. Secondly, it's possible your diet lacks in something or you just haven't found a reward that won't mess up your diet.

You can solve the first problem by frequently visualizing your future self to make it more real. The choices you make today will shape the person you will become tomorrow.

Constantly rewarding yourself with treats feels great today, but does the vision of you remaining an overweight or obese, unhealthy person, feel great, too? Each time you say "I deserve a treat" (outside of a cheat day) you also say "I'd rather get $5 today than $1000 in a few weeks." How smart is that?

If you're tempted to reward yourself on a daily basis, perhaps there's also something wrong with your diet. Maybe it lacks satisfying foods, or maybe you've trained yourself to reward yourself only with food. Come up with alternative ways to pamper yourself.

Getting a massage can be just as rewarding, if not more, than grabbing a hot dog, and it will be much more beneficial to your health. Going on a weekend trip can be a great treat for all the progress you've made the past week with your diet without reverting all of it with a few treats here and there.

Each time you want to give yourself a treat, think of non-food-related ways to reward yourself first. And if you still want to reward yourself with food, go with healthy and tasty options – a bigger portion of berries, high-quality dairy, or a whole grain bread roll.

It's My Genetics

Underlying problem: inability to acknowledge your weakness and take responsibility for your bad decisions.

Except for a few genuine conditions (hypothyroidism, Cushing's syndrome, depression) obesity has no medical reasons outside of your control. It's only a matter of a lack of self-discipline or an unwillingness to take responsibility for your current situation, instead blaming something else that has nothing to do with it.

Can genes affect to some extent whether you're obese or fit? Sure they do. Is it a legitimate excuse why you're overweight if you can do something about it? Not really. Plenty of people have been obese for a long time, yet they're fit and healthy now.

I was also overweight. I could have kept telling myself that that's how it is, that's how I'm wired. But instead, I accepted it was my responsibility to take care of my health, and not something I can't control because of X or Y.

Taking ownership of all your decisions, mistakes, successes, and failures is the first step you need to take to abandon the victim mentality and the need to rationalize everything by blaming external factors. Start today by realizing that your weight is not the outcome of things outside your control, but of very controllable things – your habits, choices, and attitude.

I Love Food Too Much

Underlying problem: being overly restrictive with your diet as well as having the wrong priorities in life.

I won't disagree – unhealthy food often tastes better than healthy food. Otherwise, it wouldn't be so hard to give it up. However, if you don't restrict yourself too much on your diet, you can still enjoy your favorite foods and try new flavors – just not as regularly as before.

For instance, you can schedule weekly or fortnightly cheat days and eat what you want and how much you want on these days. With this approach, you'll get the best of both worlds – lose weight, while still being able to indulge from time to time.

There's also a second problem with this rationalization – a lack of the right priorities. If you love food so much, prioritizing health should still be important for you. After all, how are you going to enjoy your food when you get sick? If you don't pay much attention to the nutritional value of food, and instead only focus on flavor, it's not a question of if you get sick – it's a question of when.

Indulging from time to time is fine as long as you set your priorities right and consume healthy food 80-90% of time. You can spend the remaining 10-20% enjoying whatever you want (and do it while enjoying better health). Or more likely, once you switch to eating healthy food 80-90% of the time, you will draw more pleasure out of eating what's good for you, which will be an even better outcome.

MOST COMMON WILLPOWER-RELATED PROBLEMS AND EXCUSES WHEN DIETING: QUICK RECAP

1. If you don't have time to eat healthy food, you can: stock up on frozen foods, cook in advance for a few days, or get someone else to cook for you (by using a food delivery service, going to healthy restaurants, or getting your roommate/family member to cook for you). Also, don't forget that if you don't make time for health, you'll have to make time for illness. And in the end, it will be more costly than developing healthy habits.

2. Most vegetables and fruits are cheaper than unhealthy food. They're also more filling, so it's easier to stick to a diet as you'll feel hungry less often than if you were to stick with junk food from a dollar menu.

3. Healthy food tastes bad if you make no effort to learn how to make it flavorful. Learn how to cook a few staple meals with the right combination of spices and herbs and your problem will be solved. You can also buy ready seasoning mixes so all you have to do

is cook some vegetables, and use the seasoning to have a flavorful, healthy meal.

4. If you're hungry on a diet, you should increase the amount of protein you consume. It's also possible you don't eat enough vegetables and fruits which are the most satiating foods. Don't expect to feel full if you mostly eat foods low on the Fullness Factor. It's possible you don't drink enough water and mistake thirst for hunger. Not drinking enough fluids can result in headaches or sensations similar to hunger pangs. Lastly, make sure your caloric deficit isn't too challenging.

5. If you don't believe in your ability to change, don't start a diet until you develop more willpower and self-belief. Consider introducing small positive changes in your life until you get a grasp on forming new habits. Then start tweaking your diet, and go on a full-blown one when you no longer think "I'll gain back the weight anyway."

6. If you constantly give yourself treats, you'll never reach your goal as you keep taking one step forward and two steps back. Replace your food-

related treats with something else, e.g. a massage or a trip. Also, don't forget that the rewards you give yourself today are the rewards your future self will have to pay for – in slow (or no) progress, worse health, or a total diet failure (and having to start again from scratch).

7. It's easy to blame your genes or any other external factors for your obesity. However, in 99% of cases the only person you can blame is you. Take responsibility for every single decision you take and realize that it has always been you – not the surroundings or things outside your control – that put you in the situation you are in now.

8. If you love food too much, it doesn't mean you can't lose weight. Use regular cheat days to indulge as well as try to find pleasure in eating what's good for you. With better health, you'll live longer, so you'll be able to enjoy great food for longer, too.

Chapter 6: Building a Self-Disciplined Lifestyle

Dieting is the first step to transition to a healthy lifestyle, but not the last. Many dieters make the mistake of thinking that a weight loss diet will solve all of their problems. In reality, your diet is just one aspect of becoming a healthier person.

In this chapter, we'll cover how to build a lifestyle that will develop your self-discipline in a holistic manner, letting you not only lose weight and maintain it, but also become more vibrant and happier. When you combine advice from this chapter with all of the tips from the previous chapters, you'll have everything you need to turn your life around.

Find Something to Enjoy Other than Food

And no, I'm not insinuating that food is the only thing you enjoy in life. What I mean is that the more (healthy) sources of enjoyment and achievement you introduce in your life, the more powerful of a change you'll undergo as a person. Dieting is a great start, but you can support it with several other things that will produce a synergistic effect.

Around the time I lost weight I became more interested in growing myself as a person. One thing led to another, and I became a personal growth junkie. I've noticed there are several catalysts that can multiply the beneficial effects of changing your eating habits:

1. Introducing more physical activity in your life and not doing it for the sake of exercise, but out of pure enjoyment. If I hadn't enjoyed weightlifting, I wouldn't have kept doing it. But I did, and it became one of the catalysts of change for me.

Weightlifting led to my obsession about physical excellence. I started going on long bike rides to improve my endurance. I experimented with sprinting to increase my speed. I started regularly swimming to improve my breathing. I got into tennis to master a challenging sport combining the physical and mental aspect. And most recently, I fell in love with indoor climbing.

I haven't stopped there. There are still many more activities and sports I'd like to try or practice on a regular basis. It's no longer possible for me to return to my old ways – an unhealthy diet and sedentary lifestyle. It would prevent me from doing what I love – and that's the type of a block that will guarantee a permanent change.

2. Working on your social life. We're social creatures, and other than health, nothing affects our happiness more than the people around us. As a shy person in the past, I used to dread any social interactions and occasions.

Shyness doesn't only affect your social life. It also makes it more difficult to become a healthy person. More severe cases of shyness mean that you won't take up jogging because you'll worry what others will think of you. You'll have a hard time taking up new sports, because it means meeting new people. You'll find it challenging to change your diet when you believe overweight people around you will start to question your choices while you're unable to stand up for yourself.

Boosting your self-confidence can lead to more personal growth, which in turn will help you achieve various goals in your life – including becoming a healthier person. My shyness – as bad as it was – was also of great usefulness to me, because it propelled me to explore the world of self-help books (and they've had a huge positive influence on my life).

3. Putting more focus on making your life ever bigger. Whether it's mastering a new skill, working on your career, starting a business, or moving to another place, all of these changes can dramatically affect how you perceive challenges in your life.

For instance, learning a foreign language can teach you that with enough perseverance you can master something you never thought you'd be capable of doing. Then you can carry over this discovery (and the subsequent lessons) to other areas of your life.

Each time you choose growth over security and comfort, you make your life bigger. When you become addicted to the never-ending process of improvement (also known as *kaizen* from the Japanese word meaning "improvement"), you'll make it impossible to stand still with your fitness and health levels.

Once it becomes a natural step forward to satisfy your need for self-actualization, dieting has the highest chance of success.

Make It Bigger than Just about Your Diet

There are three types of motivation that can help you achieve your goal: extrinsic, intrinsic, and prosocial motivation.

1. Extrinsic motivation is about the external rewards you'll get for achieving a certain goal – make more money, get admiration, or win a medal.

2. Intrinsic motivation is about self-actualization, learning, and pure enjoyment. You do things because you like the process of doing them – and the potential rewards don't matter as much. I doubt I would have succeeded at my own goals without the intrinsic motivation I have. The pure enjoyment and self-actualization I get through personal development for the sake of learning and improvement has helped me become a healthier person.

3. Prosocial motivation is about helping others. You do something because of altruistic reasons. Out of the three types of motivation, prosocial motivation is the strongest. Very few people would sacrifice their lives for money or admiration, while most would sacrifice for their family or best friends.

A paper by bestselling author of *Give and Take: A Revolutionary Approach to Success*, Adam Grant[xl], suggests that the desire to help others makes us go the extra mile we wouldn't otherwise go with just extrinsic and intrinsic motivation.

When you combine powerful internal motivation with prosocial motivation, you get the most effective mix to help you change your life.

Let's compare three fictional characters, Joe, Jim, and Jane, with entirely different motivations and how each affects their willpower:

Joe is all about extrinsic motivation. He wants to lose weight because more women will be interested in him. Then he'll be able to show off, and he loves when people admire him.

Jim understands that extrinsic motivation alone won't help him keep his resolutions. He wants to lose weight because he genuinely enjoys the process of self-improvement. He draws enjoyment out of fighting his temptations (and overcoming them), building his self-discipline, and becoming a better person.

Jane wants to lose weight so that she can set the right example for her children. She also wants to be around when they have their own kids, and she wants to keep up with her grandchildren.

Who's most likely to succeed? Whose stakes are so high that giving up is not an option?

Will Joe stick to his diet when he realizes that nobody cares about his appearance as much as he thought? It's almost a guarantee he'll fail at some point.

Jim is more likely to achieve success. If dieting and the process of personal growth gives him more enjoyment than the sacrifices he has to make, he'll probably achieve his goal.

However, it's Jane who's the clear winner here. It's not just about her. Her struggles have a much deeper meaning – she's doing it for her family, and you'd be hard pressed to find a more powerful motivation.

Come up with your own intrinsic and prosocial reasons why you want to lose weight and become a healthier person. They will serve you well during the period of discouragement that will undoubtedly happen at some point on your journey.

Escape Emotional Eating

Emotional eating is a common habit – not only among the obese and overweight. Stress, anger, sadness – all of these emotions can lead people to eat to make themselves feel better, and not because of physical hunger.

Boredom or discomfort can also lead to emotional eating. If it's cold and dark outside, it feels good to grab a bar of chocolate or eat a pleasantly warm pizza. If you're bored, eating can provide some entertainment or at least help you kill time.

Emotional eating doesn't always have to be bad. It's fine to celebrate a special occasion with your friends or reach for comfort food when you're feeling blue. However, if it's a regular occurrence, it can pose a challenge for your struggles to become a healthy person.

The absolute worst thing you can do to try to overcome emotional eating is to be tough on yourself. If you lack self-compassion and keep blaming yourself for eating food for emotional reasons, you'll never escape the vicious cycle.

Instead, acknowledge what you feel and don't berate yourself for emotional eating. Accept that slip-ups will happen, but as long as you keep working on ways to deal with negative emotions in a different way, you'll eventually solve your problem.

The first, most obvious way to deal with emotional eating is to remove stressors from your life. If there are certain particular situations that make you eat to calm yourself down, find ways to eliminate these situations from your life.

Is it a colleague at work? Find ways to avoid her. Is it your boss? If there's no chance she'll change, perhaps it's time to think about your priorities and find another job. Are you constantly sad and eat to lift your spirits? Seek professional help – perhaps it's depression.

If it's too difficult or impossible to get rid of certain stressors in your life, find different ways to handle your negative emotions. For instance, even brief exercise or a conversation with your friend can help you reduce stress and the urge to eat something for comfort. Getting busy – whatever the activity is – helps you forget about the stressor or at least shift a part of your attention to something else for a short while.

If you eat because you're bored, find ways to fill your time in a different way than by eating. If it's usually impulsive, wait it out. Tell yourself that you can have it in fifteen minutes. Chances are you'll forget about it before the time is up.

It's a good idea to make a list of emotional states that make you more likely to eat for comfort or to feel

better. For instance, a lack of sunlight and exercise –
especially when combined with a lack of quality sleep
– makes me more likely to eat for emotional reasons.
Even if I don't feel hungry at all, I'll keep eating
something in the hopes of feeling better.

The knowledge that this particular combination
makes me eat emotionally helps me avoid it, or at
least reduce the occurrence of it.

Eliminate Bad Habits

Getting rid of the unhealthy habits of the past can
help you transition to a more self-disciplined life. The
point is not to become a monk, but to control what
you do on a daily basis and avoid the most dangerous
behaviors that can set you back.

Here are a few of the most common bad habits
that increase the risk of falling back into old,
unhealthy behaviors:

1. Watching too much TV

There's nothing wrong with watching an episode
(or two) of your favorite TV series. The problem
starts with regular binge watching, particularly when
it's one of the primary ways to entertain yourself.

111

The main problem is how mindless we become when we watch something. If you snack on something while watching (e.g., popcorn), you're guaranteed to overeat. A distracted mind is incapable of portion control.

I get it. A great deal of the enjoyment when watching a movie is the snacks that accompany it. And there's nothing wrong with it, as long as it's not regular.

Here are a few ways to control this habit:

- only turn on the TV (or Netflix, or whatever else) when you have something specific to watch. With mindless channel surfing it's easy to spend too much time in front of TV. If you have set hours for watching TV (say, a 60-minute episode of your favorite series at 8 PM), it's easier to turn off the TV when your time is up. Distraction is the enemy of willpower, so avoid unfocused channel surfing.

- don't snack when watching TV. As mentioned before, you can mindlessly gorge on unhealthy foods and don't even realize when you consume a bag (or two) of potato chips and other unhealthy food. Keep track of how often you snack while watching TV and limit it to once a week or less.

- choose friends over TV. Whenever you're bored, don't resort to TV as your primary choice of entertainment. Instead see your friends or do something interesting and physical outside. It takes willpower to change your everyday habits, but that's precisely how you build a more self-disciplined life.

2. Not getting enough exercise

A 2012 study conducted on the impact of sitting and appetite at the Energy Metabolism Laboratory at the University of Massachusetts has shown that among the participants of the study, dramatic reduction in energy expenditure was not accompanied by reduced appetite[xli].

In other words, the participants, despite needing fewer calories to function, didn't reduce the amount of food they ate. Consequently, as the study concludes, "prolonged sitting may promote excess energy intake, leading to weight gain."

While a diet alone can help you reach your ideal weight, physical activity is what helps you achieve results faster, as well as maintain them.

A 2009 study authored by Erik Kirk and colleagues at the Department of Kinesiology & Health Education at the Southern Illinois University has shown that among sedentary, overweight young adults at high risk for developing obesity, even a minimal resistance training program (11 minutes per session) resulted in a chronic increase in energy expenditure and fat oxidation[xlii].

Last but not least, a 2012 study on neural response to pictures of food after exercise in normal-weight and obese women showed that 45-minutes of exercise produced lower brain responses to the food images and an increase in total physical activity that day[xliii].

In other words, exercise serves as an appetite-regulating mechanism as well as leads to more physical activity. It's a self-reinforcing habit that makes maintaining a healthy lifestyle so much easier

– you don't need more willpower if the first bout of exercise automatically leads to more physical activity.

With exercise – even if it's just 11 minutes a day – it's easier to maintain the proper energy balance. If you find yourself slipping back into a sedentary lifestyle, weight gain is a common side effect. After all, you burn fewer calories a day, and when you combine it with the fact you probably don't reduce your food intake despite needing fewer calories to function, you eat more than you need.

Here are a few ways to make sure you always get enough physical exercise:

- start practicing a sport you love. There's no easier way to ensure ample regular physical activity than practicing a sport you love. Few things are worse to form a habit of regular exercise than forcing people to go the gym and walk for hours on a treadmill or a similarly boring fitness machine.

Find something you like so much that you miss doing it if you don't do it for a few days. It can be cycling, tennis, martial arts, climbing, even dancing.

Whatever it is – find something enjoyable and things will take care of themselves.

- take regular breaks and move. If your work is sedentary, make sure to have at least 5 to 10 minutes away from the screen every hour. During your break, go on a brief walk or do some simple exercises like pushups, squats, or jumping jacks.

- get your friends active. Instead of always meeting with your friends for coffee, a movie, or something else that is sedentary in nature, come up with fun alternatives. Go play Frisbee, go on a walk in a park or forest, go bowling, or infect your friends with your passion for two-player sports like tennis, badminton, boxing, ping-pong, fencing, billiards, climbing, etc.

3. Not getting enough sleep

I don't think I have to tell you about all the adverse effects of not getting enough sleep. The only surprising effect you might not know about which is relevant to dieting is that according to a 2012 study at the New York Obesity Nutrition Research Center, a lack of sleep may result in enhanced appetite in men and in women because they're less full[xliv].

Please keep in mind that the study's small size (26 people) means it's only a possibility, not a certainty. However, there are other studies that point in the direction that a lack of sleep is indeed related with increased appetite and/or other behaviors that can increase the risk of obesity.

A 2013 study on the impact of sleep deprivation on food desire in the human brain has shown that the reward center of the brain of sleep-deprived people responded more strongly to images of high-calorie foods than the well-rested group[xlv].

Another study conducted at the New York Obesity Nutrition Research Center also suggests similar conclusions – a lack of sleep increases the neuronal response to unhealthy food in normal-weight individuals[xlvi].

Whatever the underlying reasons are, a lack of sleep is certainly not healthy and can affect your levels of self-discipline. Make sure to always get enough sleep, whether it's 7, 8, or 9 hours for you (depending on your level of activity). Don't forget that the quality of your sleep also plays a huge role here, so make sure your sleep is not interrupted (I share some tips in my book *How to Relax*).

4. Snacking

Never-ending snacking never ends well. If you eat just because you're used to eating something all the time, and not because of hunger, sooner or later you'll get fat. And if you've already succeeded with your diet, going back to regular snacking can lead to gaining all of the weight back.

Reconnect with your body's needs and eat primarily when you feel hungry, not to occupy yourself. Wait to eat until you feel hunger pangs, and not before.

Here are a few ways to control this habit:

- ban all types of snack food from your home. If you don't have easy access to it, you'll be less likely to eat it.

- if you absolutely can't stop snacking because your self-discipline isn't that developed yet, at least replace unhealthy snacks with healthier alternatives.

Eat regular homemade popcorn instead of microwaved popcorn. Eat pistachios instead of potato chips. Have a plate of snack fruits (kiwi, grapes, strawberries, oranges, etc.) instead of chocolate bars.

- experiment with various meal timings and the number of meals you eat a day. If you usually eat three large meals and two smaller meals a day, try to do away with the latter and eat three bigger, more satisfying meals instead. Some people (me included) just won't get satisfied with five smaller meals. I much prefer one huge, satisfying meal to three (let alone five) bird-like portions.

- occupy yourself with something. If you're focused on a certain task (and don't mistake it with the wrong zombie-like kind of focus, as in watching TV), you usually don't think about food and snacking. If you have nothing to do after work and completing all of the chores, start learning a new skill (e.g., learn a foreign language) that will shift your attention from boredom to intense focus.

5. Eating addictive foods regularly

As we've already discussed, certain types of foods are more addictive than others. While it's fine to eat them from time to time for reasons other than hunger (usually for social reasons or just for the flavor), the moment you add them to your daily menu your risk of ruining your healthy diet soars.

There's a reason why these foods are called addictive – if you develop a habit to eat them often, you won't be satisfied eating them just once in a while. For this reason, it's best to pay attention to never eat the same addictive foods for two days in a row. Ideally, you shouldn't eat them more often than once a week, if not once a month.

I can go without chocolate for weeks on end, but when I eat it once, and then eat it again the next day, suddenly I find myself unable to go without it for more than a few days. It takes at least a week or two of not eating it to forget about it. If you still don't have enough self-discipline, two or three days in a row of eating chocolate can easily turn into a destructive eating habit. From there, it's easy to see your weight go up again.

BUILDING A SELF-DISCIPLINED LIFESTYLE: QUICK RECAP

1. Diet is just one aspect of health. Losing weight and maintaining it are important pieces of the puzzle. However, to complete it, you should enrich your life with healthy habits and hobbies to make it more enjoyable. Only then will you stop being tempted to go back to your old ways – your identity will undergo such a profound change that it will no longer be possible to become the old person you used to be.

2. Three catalysts that can shake up your routine and transform your identity are:

- regular physical activity, especially if you're after excellence in a sport you practice,

- improving your social life, and especially overcoming your shyness,

- making it a habit to always look for opportunities to make your life bigger.

All of these changes can lead to a domino effect, forcing you to change the fitness/diet aspect of your life.

3. Out of the three kinds of motivation, (intrinsic, extrinsic, prosocial) prosocial motivation – doing something for the sake of helping someone else – is the most powerful and lasting motivation. If you want to build a more self-disciplined lifestyle, give it more meaning – make it not only about you, but also about others.

4. Emotional eating can make it difficult to maintain healthy habits and live a self-disciplined life.

The path toward eliminating the habit of emotional eating starts with self-compassion. Instead of beating yourself up each time you gorge on chocolate or ice cream because you were angry or sad, accept your shortcomings and move on.

Try to remove the stressors that lead to emotional eating or find alternatives to handle these negative emotions (examples include physical exercise or talking with a friend).

Don't forget that emotional eating is often impulsive. If you wait it out, it's possible you'll no longer feel the urge to eat.

5. Avoid bad habits that increase the risk of falling back into your old, unhealthy routines. Some of the most common such habits include: watching too much TV, not getting enough exercise, not getting enough sleep, snacking, and eating addictive food regularly.

6. The key to controlling the habit of watching TV is self-awareness. If you mindlessly surf channels while snacking, the habit becomes a danger to your healthy lifestyle. Whenever possible, replace TV as an entertainment with other, more physical forms of spending free time.

7. A sedentary lifestyle – even with a healthy diet – will make you regain weight. Physical activity increases your energy expenditure and reduces your appetite, thus making it easier to maintain proper energy balance (the same amount of calories in as out).

The best way to ensure you always get enough exercise is to find a sport you love. If you consider exercise a chore, it will always be challenging to get enough physical activity. If you love it, you don't need willpower at all.

8. A lack of sleep can increase hunger and decrease your willpower when trying to resist unhealthy foods. Make sure to get enough sleep, or your diet will suffer.

9. Eat when you're hungry, not out of habit. Snacking is a sure-fire way to overeat and go back to your old weight. Moreover, it's extremely difficult to control if you do it mindlessly. If you're distracted, not even a high level of willpower will help you overcome it.

If you can't stop snacking, take a step-by-step approach by replacing unhealthy snacks with healthier alternatives.

If you're ready to stop snacking, start by occupying your mind with something else whenever you get a craving to snack and experiment with various meal timings and the portions.

10. Addictive foods can lead you back into a vicious cycle of overeating. If you want to cheat from

time to time, make sure it's really "from time to time," and not regularly.

Epilogue

There's no question that dieting is challenging. Some people can achieve success the first time they try to lose weight, while others will need a few attempts before they make permanent changes. However, as long as you keep trying, you'll achieve your goal, too.

As a quick recap, please remember that:

1. Setting the right expectations and realizing that it's not about a short-term diet, but a permanent change, are crucial to success. Most people fail because they expect miracle diets to work. They don't, because you can't revert years of unhealthy habits with a few weeks of a diet. Assume you won't lose more than a pound of fat a week, and aim for a lifelong change by changing your everyday habits.

2. Cravings are passing sensations. If you can distract yourself or otherwise postpone giving in (by scheduling cheat days or cheat meals), cravings will be much easier to handle.

3. If you're satiated, it's easier to have self-discipline to resist temptations. If there's one magic trick to lose weight more easily, it's to eat many vegetables and fruits proven to be up to seven times more satiating than less healthy options like fast food.

4. If you never develop healthy and tasty alternatives, you'll always miss unhealthy foods. Become a cook – even if you only master a few simple, staple meals. If you never experience cravings for healthy food, your diet will always be challenging to maintain.

5. Recognize excuses for what they are. There are very few legitimate reasons why you can't become a healthier person by losing weight. The moment you acknowledge the responsibility for your health is the moment you can start making permanent changes.

6. Don't obsess about your diet. Find healthy hobbies and form positive habits in life to finish your transformation into a healthy, vibrant person. If you enjoy your healthy lifestyle, you'll never be tempted to go back to your old ways.

I hope that the advice from this book will help you when it comes to willpower-related challenges. After all, many problems arise because of the mental part of dieting, not because you can't bear it physically.

It's not like your body can't function with fewer calories or is so addicted to unhealthy food that you experience severe withdrawal symptoms. It only happens in your head, and the advice in this book is meant to help you overcome these mental challenges by strengthening your resolve.

If you develop the ability to overcome your ever-friendly brain trying to sell you the idea of a weak short-term reward (satisfying your craving) in exchange for a huge long-term reward (better health and overall well-being), you won't only become a successful dieter, but also greatly improve your chances of success in other areas of life.

In this sense, starting a diet and successfully changing your eating habits can have a positive transformational effect on your entire life. Looking back, you'll most likely think of it as the best thing that has ever happened to you. And that's precisely what I would love to happen to you. Give yourself a chance – sacrifices will be worth it.

Download another Book for Free

I want to thank you for buying my book and offer you another book (just as valuable as this book), *Grit: How to Keep Going When You Want to Give Up*, completely free.

Visit the link below to receive it:

http://www.profoundselfimprovement.com/selfdisciplineddieter

In *Grit*, I'll share with you exactly how to stick to your goals according to peak performers and science.

In addition to getting *Grit*, you'll also have an opportunity to get my new books for free, enter giveaways, and receive other valuable emails from me.

Again, here's the link to sign up:

http://www.profoundselfimprovement.com/selfdisciplineddieter

Could You Help?

I'd love to hear your opinion about my book. In the world of book publishing, there are few things more valuable than honest reviews from a wide variety of readers.

Your review will help other readers find out whether my book is for them. It will also help me reach more readers by increasing the visibility of my book.

About Martin Meadows

Martin Meadows is the pen name of an author who has dedicated his life to personal growth. He constantly reinvents himself by making drastic changes in his life.

Over the years, he has regularly fasted for over 40 hours, taught himself two foreign languages, lost over 30 pounds in 12 weeks, ran several businesses in various industries, took ice-cold showers and baths, lived on a small tropical island in a foreign country for several months, and wrote a 400-page long novel's worth of short stories in one month.

Yet, self-torture is not his passion. Martin likes to test his boundaries to discover how far his comfort zone goes.

His findings (based both on his personal experience and scientific studies) help him improve his life. If you're interested in pushing your limits and learning how to become the best version of yourself, you'll love Martin's works.

You can read his books here:

http://www.amazon.com/author/martinmeadows.

[i] Hall K. D., "What is the Required Energy Deficit per unit Weight Loss?" *International Journal of Obesity* 2008; 32 (3): 573–576.

[ii] http://www.fns.usda.gov/sites/default/files/Chapter2.pdf, Web., October 12th, 2015.

[iii] Hebert J. R., Patterson R. E., Gorfine M., Ebbeling C. B., St Jeor S. T., Chlebowski R. T., "Differences between estimated caloric requirements and self-reported caloric intake in the women's health initiative." *Annals of Epidemiology* 2003; 13 (9): 629–637.

[iv] *Estimated Calorie Needs per Day by Age, Gender, and Physical Activity Level*, http://www.cnpp.usda.gov/sites/default/files/usda_food_patterns/EstimatedCalorieNeedsPerDayTable.pdf, Web., October 12th, 2015.

[v] Polivy J., Herman C. P., "If at first you don't succeed. False hopes of self-change." *The American Psychologist* 2002; 57 (9): 677–689.

[vi] Lally P., van Jaarsveld C. H. M., Potts H. W. W., Wardle J. "How are habits formed: Modelling habit formation in the real world." *European Journal of Social Psychology* 2010; 40 (6): 998–1009.

[vii] Katz D. L, Meller S., "Can We Say What Diet Is Best for Health?" *Annual Review of Public Health* 2014; 35: 83–103.

[viii] http://fourhourworkweek.com/2012/07/12/how-to-lose-100-pounds/, Web., October 13th, 2015. For more information, read Ferriss T., *The 4-Hour Body: An Uncommon Guide to Rapid Fat Loss, Incredible Sex and Becoming Superhuman*, 2010.

[ix] Miller S. L., Wolfe R. R., "The danger of weight loss in the elderly." T*he Journal of Nutrition Health and Aging* 2008; 12 (7): 487–491.

[x] Rossow L. M., Fukuda D. H., Fahs C. A., Loenneke J. P., Stout J. R., "Natural bodybuilding competition preparation and recovery: a 12-month case study." *International Journal of Sports Physiology and Performance* 2013; 8 (5): 582–592.

[xi] Astrup A., Rössner S., "Lessons from obesity management programmes: greater initial weight loss improves long-term maintenance." *Obesity Reviews* 2000; 1 (1): 17–19.

[xii] Saris W. H., "Very-low-calorie diets and sustained weight loss." *Obesity Reviews* 2001; 9 (4): 295S–301S.

[xiii] Nackers L. M., Ross K. M., Perri M. G., "The association between rate of initial weight loss and long-term success in obesity treatment: does slow and steady win the race?" *International Journal of Behavioral Medicine* 2010; 17 (3): 161–167.

[xiv] Purcell K., Sumithran P., Prendergast L. A., Bouniu C. J., Delbridge E., Proietto J., "The effect of rate of weight loss on long-term weight management: a randomised controlled trial." *The Lancet Diabetes & Endocrinology* 2014; 2 (12): 954–962.

[xv] Mischel W., Ebbesen E. B., Raskoff Z. A., "Cognitive and attentional mechanisms in delay of gratification." *Journal of Personality and Social Psychology* 1972; 21 (2): 204–218.

[xvi] Shoda Y., Mischel W. Peake P. K., "Predicting Adolescent Cognitive and Self-Regulatory Competencies from Preschool Delay of Gratification: Identifying Diagnostic Conditions." *Developmental Psychology* 1990; 26 (6): 978–986.

[xvii] Loewenstein G., "Hot-cold empathy gaps and medical decision making." *Health Psychology* 2005; 24 (4): S49–S56.

[xviii] Ariely D., Loewenstein G., "The heat of the moment: the effect of sexual arousal on sexual decision making." *Journal of Behavioral Decision Making* 2006; 19: 87–98.

[xix] Dirlewanger M., di Vetta V., Guenat E., Battilana P., Seematter G., Schneiter P., Jéquier E., Tappy L., "Effects of short-term carbohydrate or fat overfeeding on energy expenditure and plasma leptin concentrations in healthy female subjects." *International Journal of Obesity and Related Metabolic Disorders: Journal of the International Association for the Study of Obesity* 2000; 24 (11): 1413–8.

[xx] Davis J. F., "Adipostatic regulation of motivation and emotion." *Discovery Medicine* 2010; 9 (48): 462–7.

[xxi] A study about the need to have a high-protein cheat day: Bray G. A., Smith S. R., de Jonge L., Xie H., Rood J., Martin C. K., Most M., Brock C., Mancuso S., Redman L. M., "Effect of dietary protein content on weight gain, energy expenditure, and body composition during overeating: a randomized controlled trial." *JAMA* 2012; 307 (1): 47–55. A study about high-carb refeeding: Dirlewanger M., di Vetta V., Guenat E., Battilana P., Seematter G., Schneiter P., Jéquier E., Tappy L., "Effects of short-term carbohydrate or fat overfeeding on energy expenditure and plasma leptin concentrations in healthy female subjects." *International Journal of Obesity and Related Metabolic Disorders: Journal of the International Association for the Study of Obesity* 2000; 24 (11): 1413–8.

[xxii] http://romanfitnesssystems.com/articles/feast-fast/, Web., October 22th, 2015.

[xxiii]
https://www.kpchr.org/research/public/News.aspx?NewsID=3, Web., November 21st, 2015.

[xxiv] Schulte E. M., Avena N. M., Gearhardt A N., "Which Foods May Be Addictive? The Roles of Processing, Fat Content, and Glycemic Load." *PLoS One* 2015; 10 (2): e0117959. Figures are available here:
http://journals.plos.org/plosone/article?id=10.1371/journal.pone.0117959.

[xxv] Clark M. J., Slavin J. L., "The effect of fiber on satiety and food intake: a systematic review." *Journal of the American College of Nutrition* 2013; 32 (3): 200–211.

[xxvi] Wasser S. P., Weis A. L., "Therapeutic Effects of Substances Occurring in Higher Basidiomycetes Mushrooms: A Modern Perspective." *Critical Reviews in Immunology* 1999; 19 (1): 65–96

[xxvii] Rolls B. J., Hetherington M., Burley V. J., "The specificity of satiety: The influence of foods of different macronutrient content on the development of satiety." *Physiology & Behavior* 1988; 43 (2): 145–153.

[xxviii] Due A., Toubro S., Skov A. R., Astrup A., "Effect of normal-fat diets, either medium or high in protein, on body weight in overweight subjects: a randomised 1-year trial." *International Journal of Obesity* 2004; 28: 1283–1290.

[xxix] Paddon-Jones D., Westman E., Mattes R. D., Wolfe R. R., Astrup A., Westerterp-Plantenga M., "Protein, weight management, and satiety." *The American Journal of Clinical Nutrition* 2008; 87 (5): 1558S–1561S.

[xxx] Noakes M., "The role of protein in weight management." *Asia Pacific Journal of Clinical Nutrition* 2008; 17 Suppl 1: 169–171.

[xxxi] You can estimate your body fat percentage and lean body mass by using a simple US Navy formula, available here: http://rippedbody.jp/how-calculate-body-fat-percentage/ (or just google "us navy body fat calculator").

[xxxii] Tsutsumi R., Tsutsumi Y. M., "Peptides and Proteins in Whey and Their Benefits for Human Health." *Austin Journal of Nutrition and Food Sciences* 2014; 1 (1): 1002.

[xxxiii] Pal S., Ellis V, Dhaliwal S., "Effects of whey protein isolate on body composition, lipids, insulin and glucose in overweight and obese individuals." *The British Journal of Nutrition* 2010; 104 (5): 716–23.

[xxxiv] Hall W. L., Millward D. J., Long S. J., Morgan L. M., "Casein and whey exert different effects on plasma amino acid profiles, gastrointestinal hormone secretion and appetite." *The British Journal of Nutrition* 2003; 89 (2): 239–248.

[xxxv] Hursel R., van der Zee L., Westerterp-Plantenga M. S., "Effects of a breakfast yoghurt, with additional total whey protein or caseinomacropeptide-depleted alpha-lactalbumin-enriched whey protein, on diet-induced thermogenesis and appetite suppression." *The British Journal of Nutrition* 2010; 103 (5): 775–780.

[xxxvi] Madzima T. A., Panton L. B., Fretti S. K., Kinsey A. W., Ormsbee M. J. "Night-time consumption of protein or carbohydrate results in increased morning resting energy

expenditure in active college-aged men." *The British Journal of Nutrition* 2014; 111 (1): 71–77.

[xxxvii] http://nutritiondata.self.com/topics/fullness-factor, Web., October 27th, 2015.

[xxxviii]

http://pbhfoundation.org/pdfs/pub_sec/webinars/Pegg_Webinar_April_2014_FINAL.pdf, Web., October 30h, 2015.

[xxxix] Rao M., Afshin A., Singh G., Mozzafarian D. "Do healthier foods and diet patterns cost more than less healthy options? A systematic review and meta-analysis." *BMJ Open* 2013; 3.

[xl] Grant A. M. "Does Intrinsic Motivation Fuel the Prosocial Fire? Motivational Synergy in Predicting Persistence, Performance, and Productivity." *Journal of Applied Psychology* 2008; 93 (1): 48–58.

[xli] Granados K., Stephens B. R., Malin S. K., Zderic T. W., Hamilton M. T., Braun B., "*Appetite regulation in response to sitting and energy imbalance.*" *Applied Physiology, Nutrition, and Metabolism* 2012, 37 (2): 323–333.

[xlii] Kirk E. P., Donnelly J. E., Smith B. K., Honas J., Lecheminant J. D., Bailey B. W., Jacobsen D. J., Washburn R. A., "Minimal resistance training improves daily energy expenditure and fat oxidation." *Medicine and Science in Sports and Exercise* 2009; 41 (5): 1122–9.

[xliii] Hanlon B., Larson M. J., Bailey B. W., LeCheminant J. D., "Neural response to pictures of food after exercise in normal-weight and obese women." *Medicine and Science in Sports and Exercise* 2012; 44 (10): 1864–70.

[xliv] St-Onge M. P., O'Keeffe M., Roberts A. L., RoyChoudhury A., Laferrère B., "Short Sleep Duration, Glucose Dysregulation and Hormonal Regulation of Appetite in Men and Women." *SLEEP* 2012; 35 (11): 1503–1510.

[xlv] Greer M. S., Goldstein A. N., Walker M. P., "The impact of sleep deprivation on food desire in the human brain." *Nature Communications* 2013; 4: 2259.

[xlvi] St-Onge M. P., Wolfe S., Sy M., Shechter A., Hirsch J., "Sleep restriction increases the neuronal response to unhealthy

food in normal-weight individuals." *International Journal of Obesity London* 2014; 38 (3): 411–416.

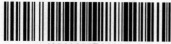

49766625R00089

Made in the USA
San Bernardino, CA
04 June 2017